AF556008

Canine Dermatopathology

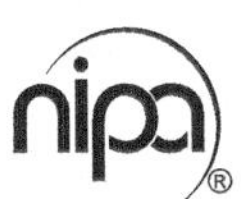

NIPA® GENX ELECTRONIC RESOURCES & SOLUTIONS P. LTD.
New Delhi-110 034

About the Authors

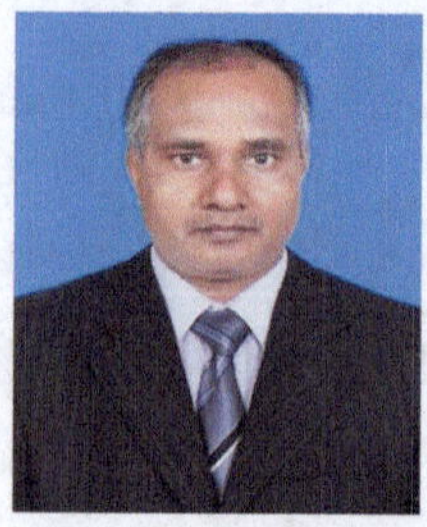

Dr. N. Pazhanivel, M.V.Sc., Ph.D., M.A. (Public Administration), PGDEVP., Diplomate ICVP., FASAW, ICMR DHR IF, and Professor of Pathology, Madras Veterinary College, Chennai-600 007. His areas of research include oncology, avian oncogenic viruses, avian pathology, cytopathology, histopathology and toxicopathology. He has published 298 research articles (International -62; National-236). He has presented 293 research papers (International-91; National-202). He has received 48 awards. He has published 3 books and 40 book chapters. He has completed 5 projects and currently 2 projects are handling. He has completed Post- Doctoral Fellowship Research Training at Pennsylvania State University, USA in 2020. At present, he is the Secretary, Indian College of Veterinary Pathologists (ICVP) from 2020.

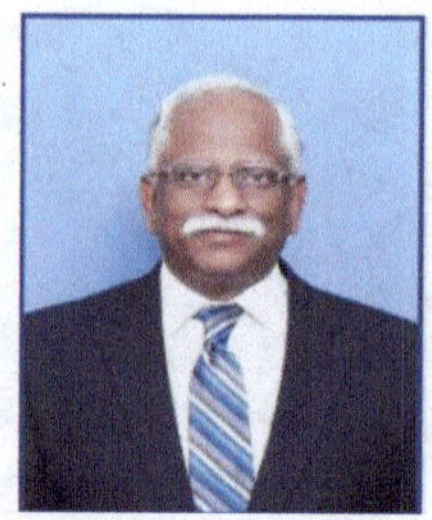

Dr. C. Balachandran was born on 28.07.1957 in Mannargudi town of Tiruvarur District, Tamil Nadu. He obtained B.V.Sc., M.V.Sc. and Ph.D. (Veterinary Pathology) degrees from Madras Veterinary College. He is PG Diploma Holder in Agricultural Journalism and Ethno Veterinary Practices,. He started his career at Namakkal in 1980 and promoted as Associate Professor in 1988 and Professor in 1996. He served as Vice-Chancellor of Tamil Nadu Veterinary and Animal Sciences University (TANUVAS) for three years from 09-04-2018.He also served as Registrar of TANUVAS and as the Dean, Madras Veterinary College. He has published about 400 scientific articles including 73 articles in International journals. He was instrumental in introducing cytological diagnosis of disease in animals. His areas of research interests are avian diseases, cytology, cancer biology and indigenous medicinal effects. He has published about 50 popular articles. He served as Editor, Kalnadai Kathir, a TANUVAS Tamil Popular Magazine. He is a Charter member of Indian College of Veterinary Pathologists and Diplomate of Indian College of Veterinary Pathologists. He has about 90 awards to his credit. Notable Awards: University gold medal for the best thesis in avian diseases, Fellow of FAO, IAVP, National Academy of Veterinary Sciences and Academy of Science for Animal Welfare, Tamil Nadu State Scientist Award.

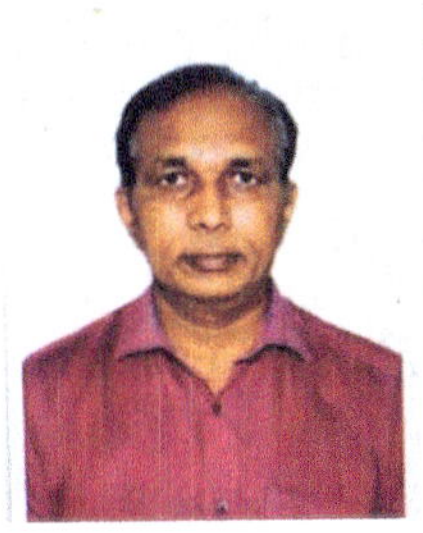

Dr. Ganne Venkata Sudhakar Rao is currently working as Professor and Head, Department of Veterinary Pathology, Madras Veterinary College, of Tamil Nadu Veterinary and Animal Sciences University (TANUVAS), Chennai - 600 007. He was born on 12.06.1964 in Thotlavalluru, Krishna District, Andhra Pradesh. He obtained B.V.Sc.& AH degree from College of Veterinary Science, APAU, Tirupati (1986), M.V.Sc. in Veterinary Pathology from Madras Veterinary College (MVC), Tamil Nadu Agricultural University (TNAU) 1989 and Ph.D. in Veterinary Pathology from TANUVAS (1997). He started his career as Assistant Professor at Veterinary College and Research Institute (VCRI) Namakkal in 1990. He was the recipient of the Associate ship of the National Academy of Sciences, United States of America and worked at the NIOSH – CDC from 2000 to 2002. He worked as Associate Professor at MVC from 2002 to 2005 and as Associate Professor and Head at the Veterinary University Training and Research Centre, Karur in 2005 and at MVC from 2006 to 2009. He worked as Professor at MVC from 2009 to 2012 and 2015 to 2017 and as Professor and Head at Farmers Training Centre, Kancheepuram from 2012 to 2015. He has published several articles in scientific and popular journals and prepared teaching manuals. He was actively involved in conducting various scientific seminars and training programs for veterinarians. He has guided several students for M.V.Sc and Ph.D in Veterinary Pathology.

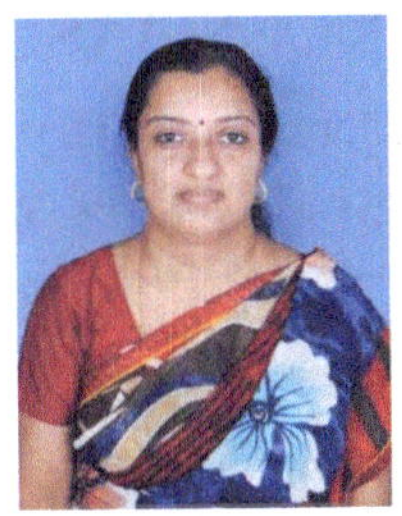

Dr. D. Sumathi, PhD., PGDRM is currently working as Professor at Department of Veterinary Clinical Medicine, Veterinary College and Research Institute, Namakkal. She has 18 years of teaching experience, 11 years of research experience and 13 years of extension experience. Her areas of specialization are Small Animal Internal Medicine (Gastroenterology & Hepatology), Small Animal Ultrasonography, Small Animal Critical Care and Small Animal Dermatology. She has completed her Postgraduate diploma in Regenerative Medicine from Madras Veterinary College. She has completed 3 research schemes as Co-Principal Investigator. She has completed a student TNSCST project from 2014-2015. She has published 30 research papers. She has received 11 best clinical presentation awards at national level. She has developed four E-courses. She was involved in UG teaching for 12 years and PG Teaching for 6 Years. She has acted as chairman for 4 postgraduate students. She has acted as chairman for 15 postgraduate diploma students in 3 subjects from 2011 to 2015. She was co-organizing Secretary in International workshop on working Dogs during 2014. She was course director for ICAR CAFT (1 completed each in 2014 & 2015). She has acted as Nodal Officer for Indian Immunological Training in the year 2014. She was co-coordinator in ECM and DUS PG Diploma Program.

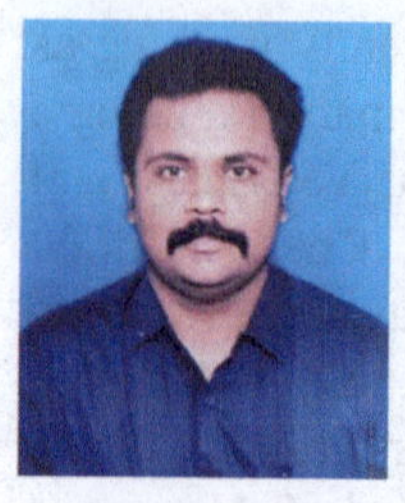

Dr. P. C. Prabu, is a Veterinary Pathologist currently working as Assistant Professor in the Department of Veterinary Pathology, VCRI, Orathanadu, Tamil Nadu Veterinary & Animal Sciences University. He has 15 years of expertise in Laboratory Animal Management and Animal welfare regulations. He has served as Laboratory Animal Veterinarian under DST Animal Facility Project and was involved in the establishment of the Laboratory Animal Facility including the Transgenic facility at the Central Animal Facility, SASTRA University including CPCSEA registration of the facility and maintenance of CPCSEA registration for the purpose of experimentation, breeding and sales of laboratory animals. He has also established the Histopathology and Clinical Pathology by 2008 exclusively for laboratory animals. Since then, he has been primarily, a lab animal Veterinarian / Study director / Pathologist and was involved in the conduct of 300 + laboratory animal experiments including toxicology and pharmacology studies.

He has been the Member Secretary of the IAEC, SASTRA and served as IAEC member as Veterinarian Incharge of the Facility for 11 years and have conducted 33 IAEC meetings. In 2014, he got the facility certified under NABL for Biological Testing. He has more than 14 years of experience in preclinical research at various levels as Lab Animal Veterinarian, Study Pathologist, Study director and Deputy Technical Manager. At the Madras Veterinary College, TANUVAS, he was involved in the laboratory animal experiments conducted by the postgraduate and doctoral students of the Department of Veterinary Pathology, MVC, TANUVAS.

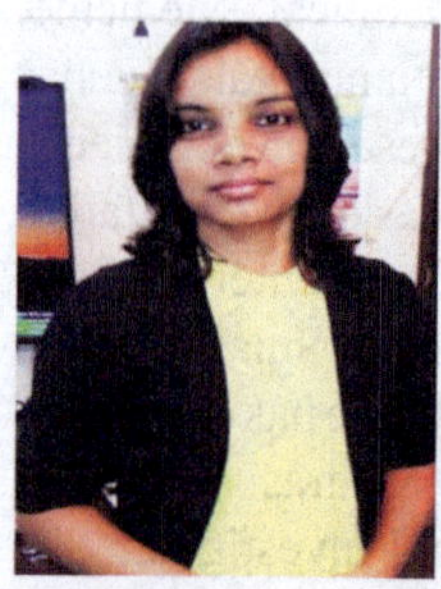

Dr. R. Saahithya, M.V.Sc., Assistant Professor of Veterinary Pathology, Veterinary College and Research Institute, Salem-636 112. She has obtained B.V.Sc., and M.V.Sc. (Veterinary Pathology) degrees from Madras Veterinary College, Chennai – 600 007 during 2013 and 2018 respectively. She did her externship at Virginia Maryland Regional College of Veterinary Medicine, Virginia Tech, USA during 2013. She was awarded with 8 gold medals and secured university third in undergraduate degree. She was awarded with 5 gold medals and secured university first in postgraduate degree in Veterinary Pathology. She was the best female outgoing student in both UG and PG curriculum in the University. She has cleared ICAR NET exam in 2018.

She started her career when she was awarded with Graduate Assistantship to serve the University from 2014. Her postgraduate research work was related to Experimental Oncology. She has published 30 scientific articles in peer reviewed journals. She has been awarded with 5 awards for best presentation at various conferences.

Canine Dermatopathology
A Colour Atlas

N. Pazhanivel
Professor
Department of Veterinary Pathology
Madras Veterinary College, Chennai – 600 007, Tamil Nadu, India

C. Balachandran
Former Vice Chancellor
Tamil Nadu Veterinary and Animal Sciences University
Madhavaram Milk Colony, Chennai-600 051, Tamil Nadu, India

Ganne Venkata Sudhakar Rao
Professor and Head
Department of Veterinary Pathology
Madras Veterinary College, Chennai-600 007, Tamil Nadu, India

D. Sumathi
Professor
Department of Veterinary Clinical Medicine
Madras Veterinary College
Chennai-600 007, Tamil Nadu, India

P.C. Prabu
Assistant Professor
Department of Veterinary Pathology
Veterinary College & Research Institute, Orathanadu -614 625

R. Saahithya
Assistant Professor
Department of Veterinary Pathology
Veterinary College and Research Institute
Salem-636 112

NIPA® GENX ELECTRONIC RESOURCES & SOLUTIONS P. LTD.
New Delhi-110 034

NIPA® GENX ELECTRONIC RESOURCES & SOLUTIONS P. LTD.

101,103, Vikas Surya Plaza, CU Block
L.S.C.Market, Pitam Pura, New Delhi-110 034
Ph : +91 11 27341616, 27341717, 27341718
E-mail: newindiapublishingagency@gmail.com
www: www.nipabooks.com

For customer assistance, please contact
Phone: + 91-11-27 34 17 17
Fax: + 91-11- 27 34 16 16

ISBN: 978-93-95763-80-6

Composed and Designed by NIPA®.

Preface

Dermatology constitutes a large percentage of the daily caseload in small animal practice and can represent a challenge for the Veterinarian as many different diseases have similar presenting signs. Thus, a solid understanding of how to approach a dermatological case logically and sequentially is essential for a successful outcome.

Dermatological disorders are one of the most common health problems and difficult to cure in pet animals especially in dogs. Pet owners are fond of healthy shiny skin coat in dogs. But, most of the time, dogs are commonly affected with ecto/endoparasitic infestations followed by contact allergens, physical causes, radiation, infectious causes (bacterial, viral, fungal infections), immunological causes, nutritional / metabolic disorders and endocrine imbalance etiologies.

Majority of the dermatological cases seen in veterinary practice can be successfully managed when the diagnostic aspect pertaining to the secondary infections are taken care of. The skin being the largest organ of the body having multiple functions such as sensory perception, thermoregulation, immune protection, vitamin D production and safeguards the animal and the environment. The initial diagnostic approach for skin diseases depends on obtaining detailed history with thorough physical and dermatological examination. The evaluation offers precious information and guides the investigative process. Specific tests should be performed in advanced cases.

Skin scrapings, trichogram, fungal and bacterial culture, cytological evaluation and skin biopsy are important diagnostic techniques in dermatology. Cytology is the highly efficient and valuable exam to evaluate a lesion rapidly, after which it becomes possible to establish the next step in the diagnostic approach. Histopathology associated with clinical findings leads to a definitive diagnosis. Skin biopsy is recommended in unusual lesions like neoplastic nodules, conditions with poor response to previous therapy and also to exclude differential diagnoses.

Recognition of basic distribution patterns gives us a practical approach to most of the common skin diseases in dogs. The knowledge – update of various dermatological disorders in dogs will pave the way for correct and early diagnosis and treatment to the dogs by using gross, cytological and histopathological lesions.

In this regard, this book deals with Diagnosis of Dermatological Conditions of Dogs with reference to cytology, gross morphology, histopathology and immunohistochemistry.

This book caters to the needs of Veterinarians (Clinicians, students, faculties) as a ready reckoner and as an educational tool to learn and differentially diagnose the various skin conditions in dogs.

Chennai **Authors**

Contents

Cutaneous Neoplasm – Epithelial Tumors

Cutaneous Neoplasm – Round Cell Tumors

List of Figures

Disorders of Infectious and Non-Infectious Origin

1

Acral Lick Dermatitis (Lick granuloma)

Etiology

Acral lick dermatitis is usually observed on extremities of dogs and the probable etiology is persistent licking. It is also caused due to self-trauma or mutilation.

Cytology

Cytology reveals the presence of intact neutrophils and bipolar organisms (Figure 1).

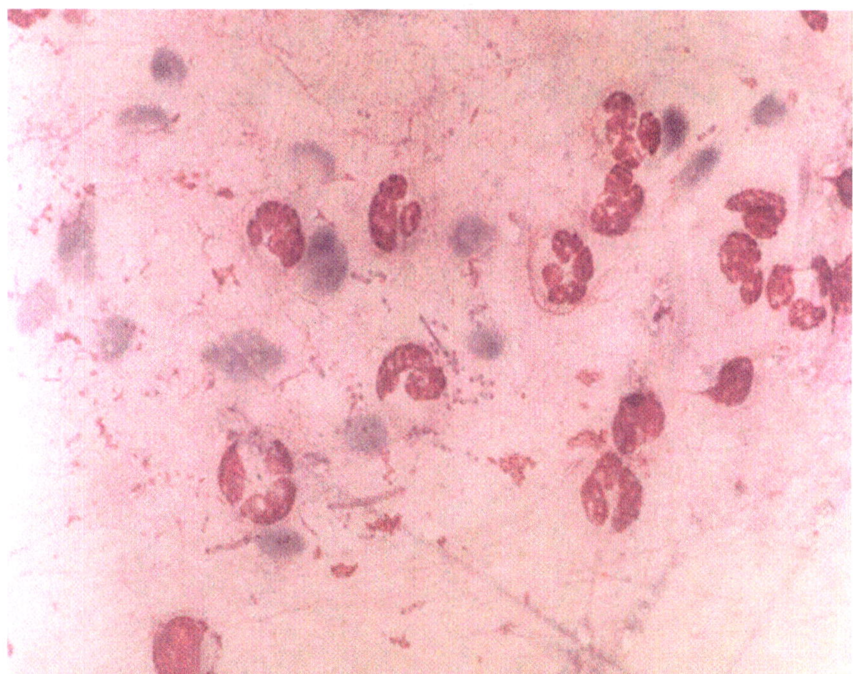

Fig. 1: Acral lick dermatitis – Cytology - Presence of intact neutrophils and bipolars Leishman-Giemsa stain 100X

Gross pathology

On gross examination, well circumscribed firm alopecic plaques and ulcerated lesions are found (Figure 2). It is usually solitary, oval and varied in diameter from two to six cm.

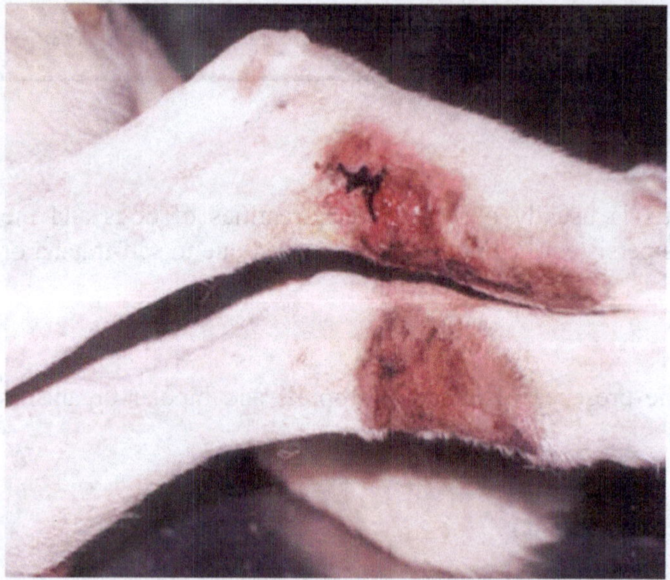

Fig. 2: Acral lick dermatitis - Erythema and ulceration

Histopathology

The condition is characterized by compact hyperkeratosis, parakeratosis, epidermal hyperplasia and vertical streaking fibrosis.

2

Atopic Dermatitis

Etiology

Atopic dermatitis is genetically predisposed to allergic skin disease. It consists of atopy and hereditary cause to produce IgE mediated allergic reaction to environmental allergens.

Immunohistochemistry reveals the presence of Langerhans cell proliferation and strong positive expression of IgE in skin tissue sections.

Gross pathology

There will be presence of erythema, excoriation and self-trauma induced alopecia.

Histopathology

Atopic dermatitis is characterized by multifocal irregular acanthosis and multifocal, mild, dermal mononuclear cell infiltration (Figure 3) with severe laminar fibrosis.

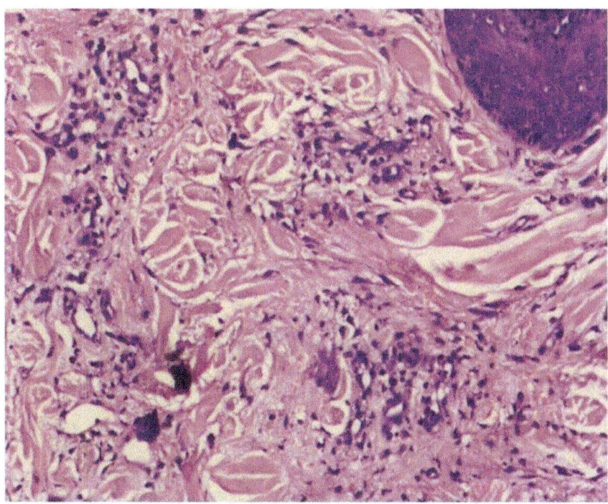

Fig. 3: Atopic dermatitis - Multifocal mild dermal mononuclear cell infiltration H&E Bar = 20µm

3

Superficial Pyoderma

Etiology

Superficial pyoderma usually occurs in the epidermis and upper infundibulum of the hair follicle. It usually heals without scar formation and commonly caused by Gram positive cocci Staphylococcus spp., particularly exfoliative toxin of this species.

Gross pathology

External lesions reveal erythema, alopecia, macules (Figure 4), papules, pustules, crusts and peripheral collarettes in the epidermis.

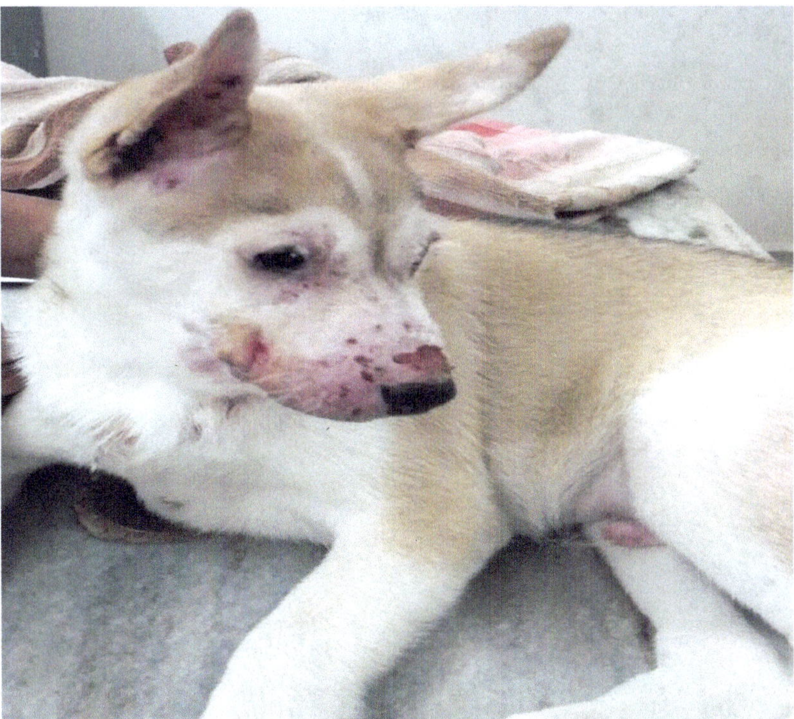

Fig. 4: Superficial pyoderma - Erythema and macules

Histopathology

Superficial pyoderma is characterized by superficial suppurative luminal folliculitis, spongiotic (Figure 5) pustule, presence of Gram-positive cocci within the superficial layers of the keratin. There is presence of granular basophilic cell debris called as Dunstan 's blue line.

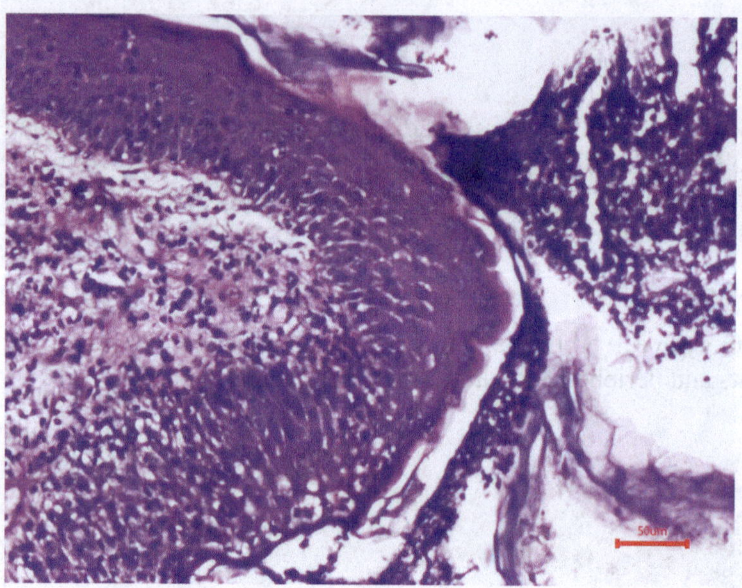

Fig. 5: Superficial pyoderma - Presence of mild spongiosis and pustule H&E Bar=50 μm

4

Superficial Pustular Dermatitis

Etiology

It is caused by *Staphylococci* spp- characterized by superficial pyoderma in dogs. It is mainly due to exfoliative toxins of *S. aureus*.

Gross pathology

The lesion reveals cutaneous exfoliation, vesicles, pustules (Figure 6) and crust.

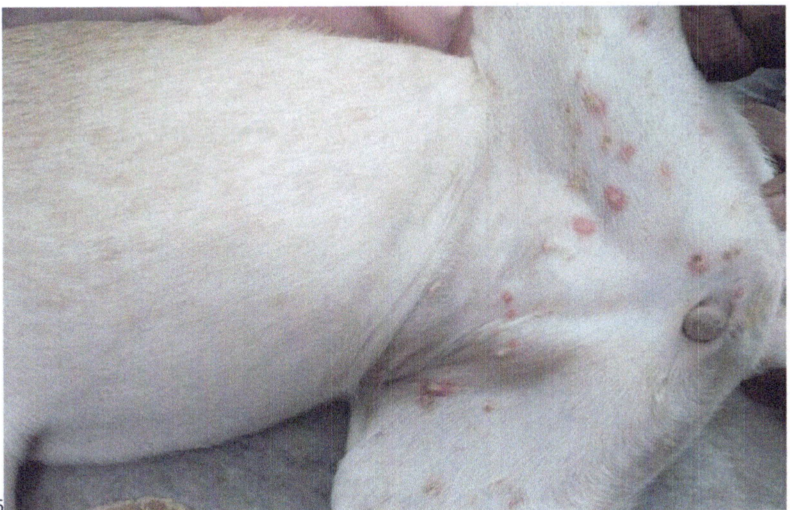

Fig. 6: Superficial pustular dermatitis

Histopathology

There is presence of pustular dermatitis with degenerative and necrotic neutrophils (Figure 7 & 8) and *Staphylococcus* spp. organisms in between the stratum corneum and stratum granulosum.

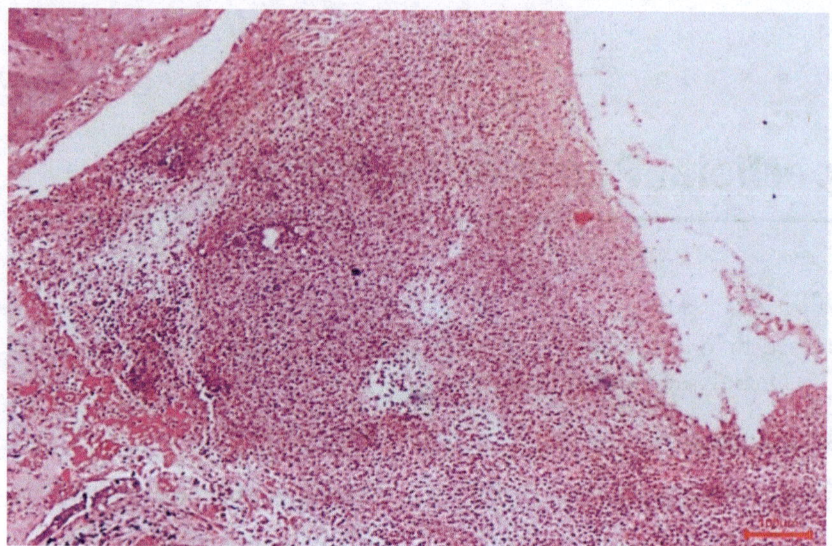

Fig. 7: Superficial pustular dermatitis H&E Bar=100 μm

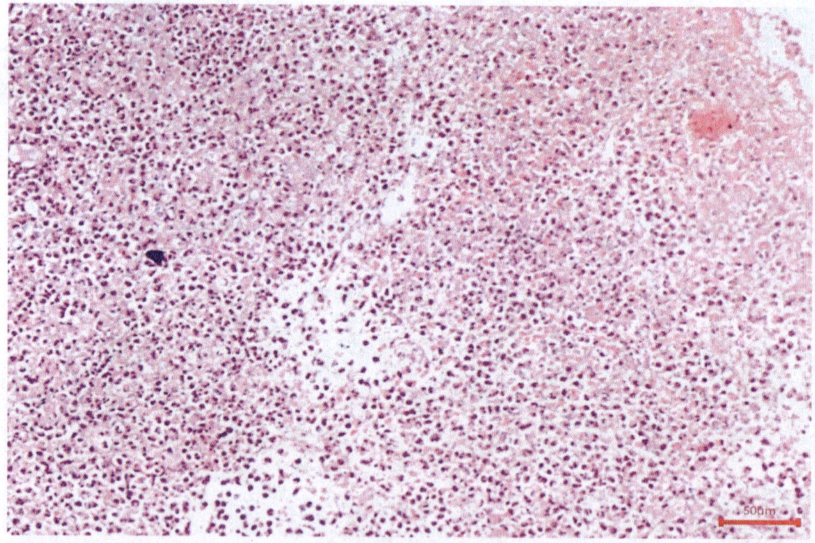

Fig. 8: Superficial pustular dermatitis - Presence of degenerative and necrotic neutrophils H&E Bar=50 μm

5

Bacterial Granulomatous Dermatitis (Bacterial granuloma)

Etiology

The condition is usually caused by implantation of low virulent saprophytic bacteria due to traumatic injury. These organisms stimulate cell mediated immune response by persistence of antigen in the tissue.

Cytology

Cytological examination reveals the presence of neutrophils and multinucleated cells (Figure 9) .

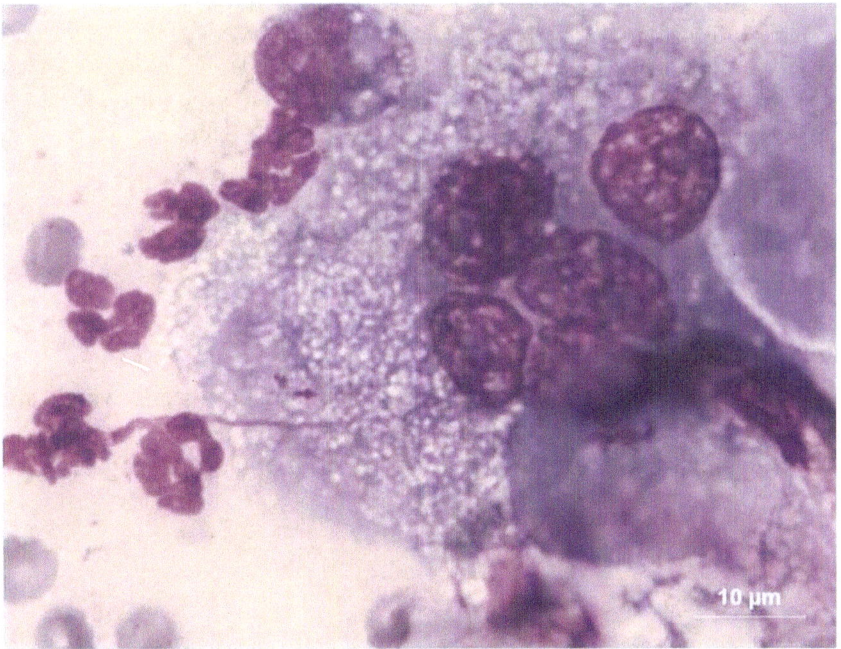

Fig. 9: Bacterial granuloma- Cytology - Chronic active inflammation characterized by the presence of neutrophils and multinucleated cell L&G Bar=10 µm

Gross pathology

Gross lesions are slowly enlarging solitary (Figure 10) to multiple nodules with or without drainage. Sometimes, it can be drained through skin surface via sinuses.

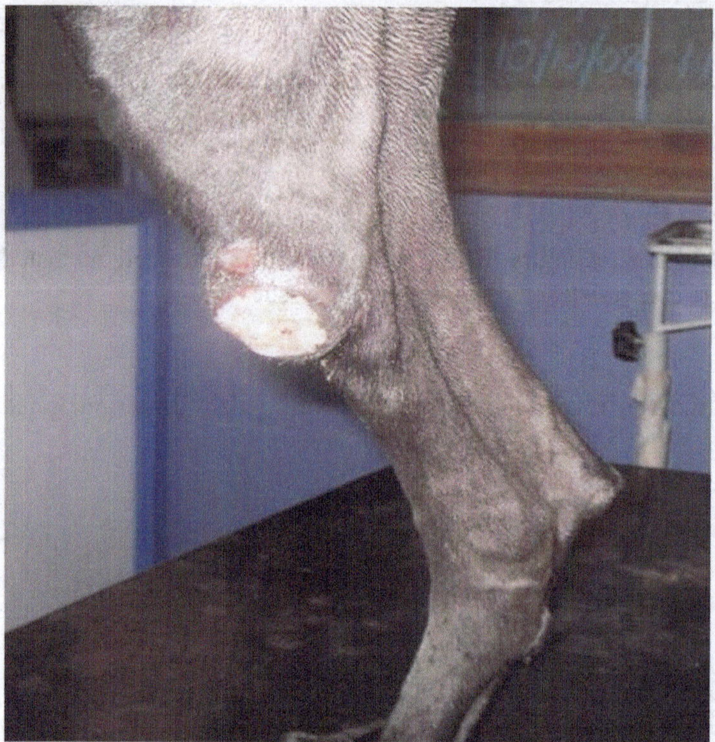

Fig. 10: Bacterial granuloma - Solitary nodule

Histopathology

This condition reveals mixed population of inflammatory cells which are composed of neutrophils, macrophages and multinucleated giant cells. The lesion also comprises caseous necrosis and bacterial organisms (Figure 11 & 12).

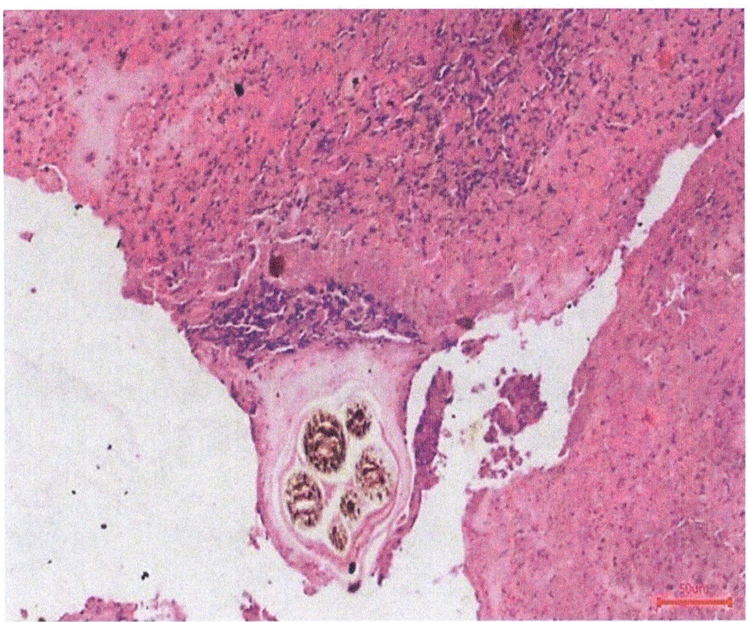

Fig.11: Bacterial granuloma H&E Bar=50 μm

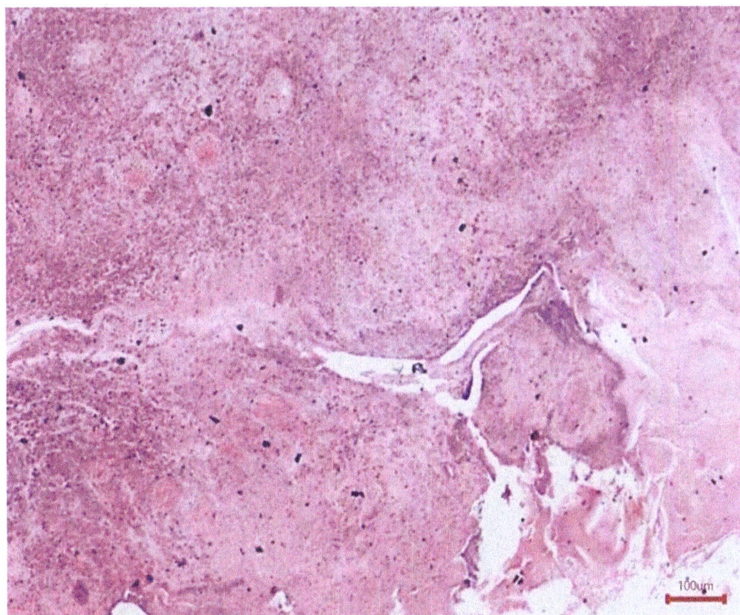

Fig. 12: Bacterial granuloma - Presence of neutrophils, macrophages, multinucleated giant cells, caseous necrosis and bacterial organisms H&E Bar=100 μm

6

Mycobacterial Granuloma

Etiology

The condition is characterized by formation of granuloma to pyogranulomatous dermatitis with paniculitis. The causative organism is normally present in the macrophage which may be *Mycobacterium tuberculosis, M. bovis* and *M. microti*.

Gross pathology

There is presence of single to multifocal coalescing nodules with draining sinuses in the dermis and subcutaneous tissue of the skin.

Histopathology

It is characterized by pyogranuloma consisting of neutrophils and macrophages with bacterial colonies. In addition, the presence of pink coloured acid fast organisms demonstrated by Ziehl - Neelsen technique is the definitive diagnosis for tuberculosis.

7

Hook Worm Dermatitis

Synonym – Cutaneous ancylostomiasis

Etiology

Hook worm dermatitis is uncommon or rare skin disease due to larval migration of the normal life cycle of *Ancylostoma braziliensis* and *Ancylostoma caninum*. It is mainly due to hypersensitive reactions against migrating third stage larvae in the distal extremities.

Gross pathology

Gross lesion reveals early erythema, erythematous papules, swelling, alopecia and lichenification.

Histopathology

Histopathologically, there will be acanthosis, erosion, multifocal spongiosis, parakeratosis and serosal crust. In the dermis, there will be mild to moderate superficial perivascular and interstitial eosinophilic infiltration. The migratory larva produces tracts characterized by linear accumulations of neutrophils and eosinophils in the epidermis to dermis. However, the larvae are rarely seen in the sections.

8

Flea Bite Hypersensitivity (Canine Flea Allergic Dermatitis, Flea Bite Dermatitis)

The condition is one of the most common pruritic skin disease caused by hypersensitivity reaction to the flea salivary antigens. Type I immediate hypersensitivity, type II delayed hypersensitivity and cutaneous basophil hypersensitivity to the flea salivary antigens have been recorded. Late phase IgG mediated reaction also caused in this condition. It occurs in dogs mostly between 1 and 3 years of age.

Clinical signs

The major clinical sign is pruritus and it occurs in any breed.

Gross pathology

Gross examination reveals alopecia, lichenification, hyperpigmentation, erythema and papules which are bilaterally symmetrical (Figure 13).

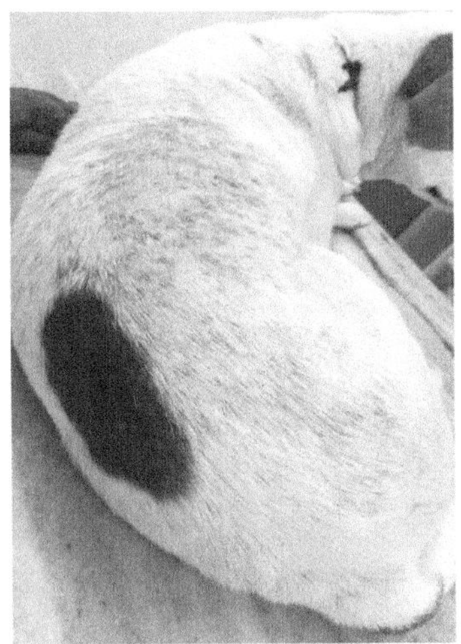

Fig. 13: Flea bite dermatitis – Bilateral erythema and papules

Histopathology

Histopathologically, there will be irregular acanthosis, patchy spongiosis, patchy parakeratosis and serocellular crust. Superficial perivascular eosinophil and mononuclear cell infiltration is also seen.

9

Pemphigus Foliaceous

Etiology

Pemphigus foliaceous is a bullous autoimmune skin disease of canines affecting epidermis and hair follicles. The recorded targeted auto-antigen in canine pemphigus foliaceous is desmoglein 1 (Dsg 1). This auto-antibody binds to Dsg 1 which is a prominent component of desmosome in the superficial layer of epidermis and hair follicle. It may be due to loss of intercellular cohesion leading to acantholysis followed by formation of superficial vesicles and bullae. The common sites for the development of pemphigus in dogs are dorsal lateral muzzle, temporal, planum nasale, pinnae, periorbital skin and paw pads.

Cytology

Cytological examination reveals the presence of acantholytic keratinocytes with neutrophils (Figure 14).

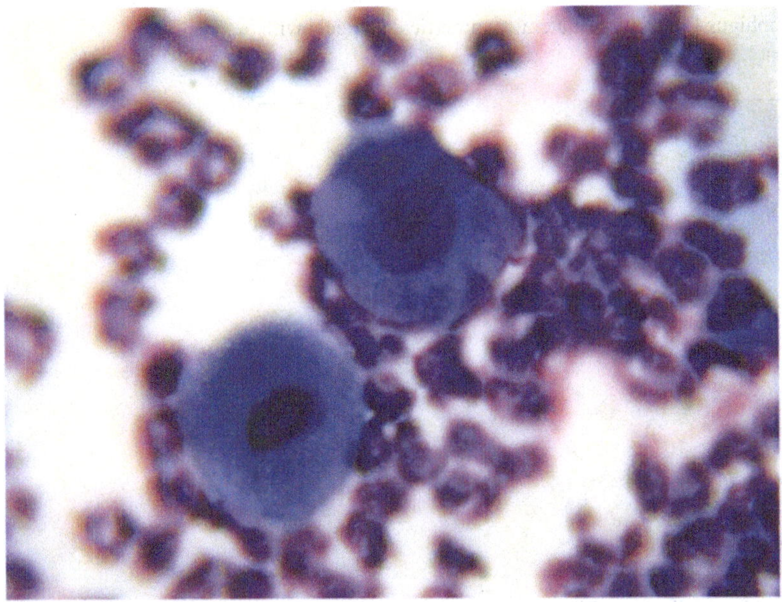

Fig. 14: Presence of acantholytic keratinocytes with neutrophils L&G 40X

Gross pathology

Gross lesions reveal the presence of superficial pustules or vesiculo pustules (wave - like pattern), keratinous crust formation in a wave - like pattern. The pustules are larger in size measuring about 2-6 mm in diameter and varied colors from translucent to grey white and yellow. Coalescence of pustules is also possible. This is frequently observed in multiple hair follicles. Pustules later form thick crust with marked exfoliation. Bilateral symmetrical alopecia and adherent crust (Figure 15) with erythema (Figure 16) are also observed.

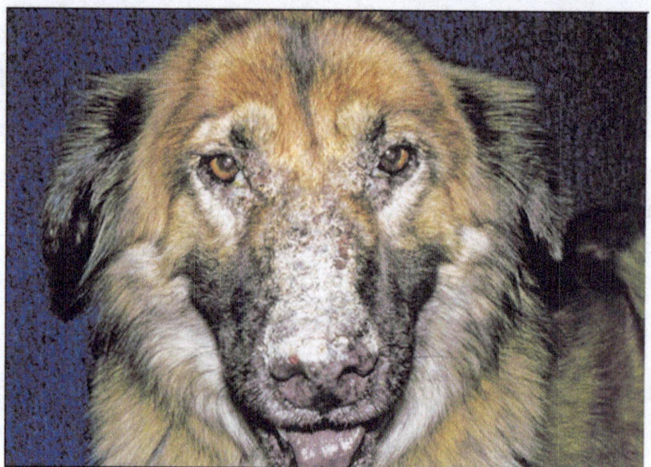

Fig. 15: Pemphigus foliaceus - Bilateral symmetrical alopecia with adherent crust

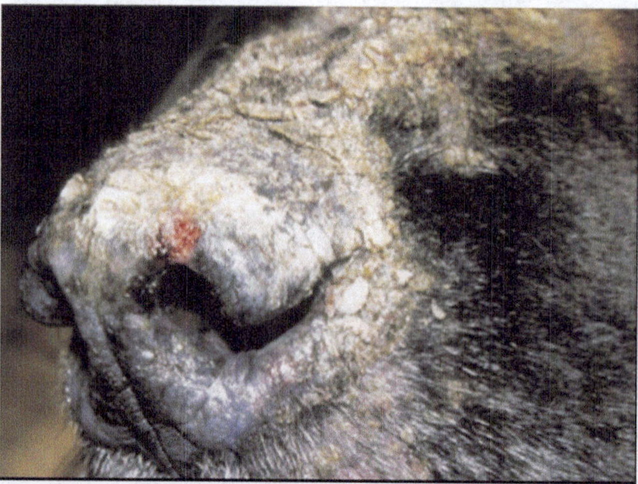

Fig. 16: Pemphigus foliaceus - Bilateral symmetrical alopecia with adherent crust and erythema (lateral view)

Histopathology

Microscopical examination reveals the presence of subcorneal pustules with acantholytic cells (Figure 17 & 18). These acantholytic cells are either freely floating or adhered to the roof of the pustule. Pustule consists of neutrophils and most of the times eosinophils. Individualized rounded bright eosinophilic acantholytic keratinocytes are seen in the pustules as small to large numbers.

Immunohistochemical testing with IgG will give positive result for pemphigus foliaceous.

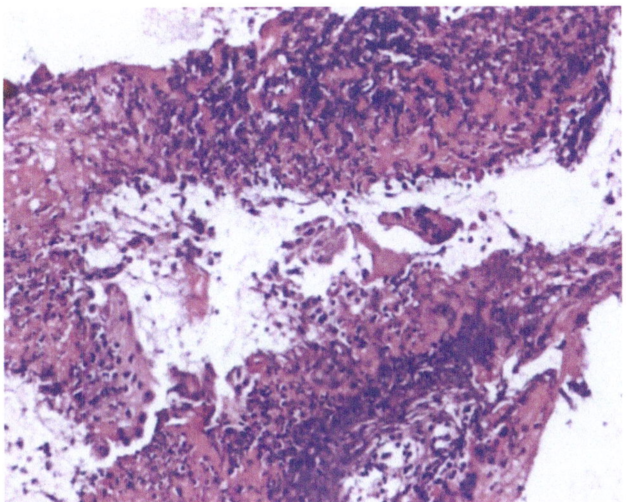

Fig. 17: Pustule containing acantholytic cells H&E 10x

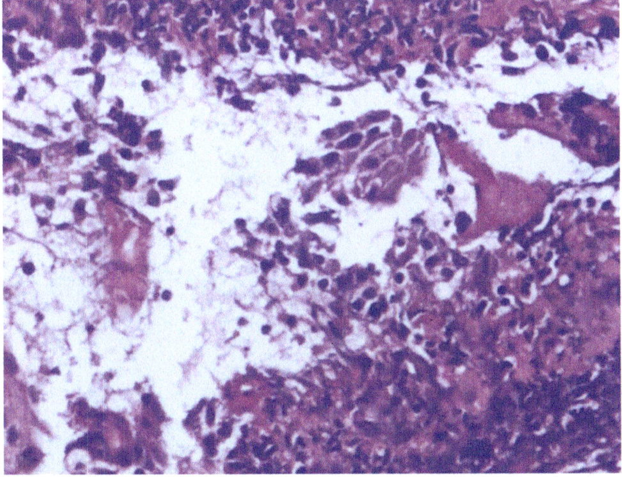

Fig. 18: Pustule containing acantholytic cells H&E 20x

10

Dysplastic Diseases of Adnexae

The disease is characterized by irregular growth and development of hair follicles and associated glands.

Sebaceous gland hyperplasia: It is a rare disease of dogs characterized by high hair coat and underlying skin, greasiness and in mainly due to excessive greasiness followed by clumping of the hair coat.

Gross pathology

Gross lesions reveals increase in size and number of sebaceous gland lobules.

Histopathology

Microscopically normal to mild acanthotic epidermis with uniform enlarged sebaceous gland and increase in the number of sebaceous gland are seen (Figure 19).

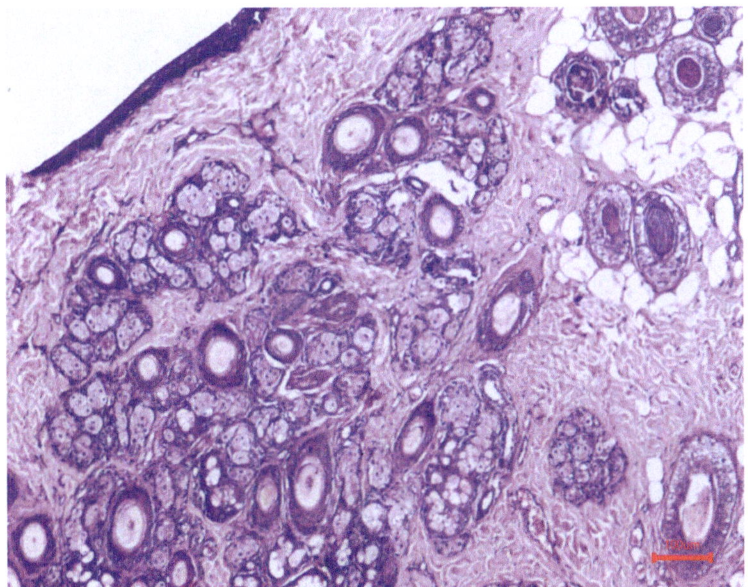

Fig. 19: Increase in number of sebaceous glands H&E Bar = 100 μm

11

Dysplastic Diseases of Adnexae

It is characterized by irregular growth and development of hair follicles and associated glands.

Sweat gland hyperplasia: It is characterized by increased number of sweat gland epithelial cells (Figure 20) and mostly this occurs due to food allergy.

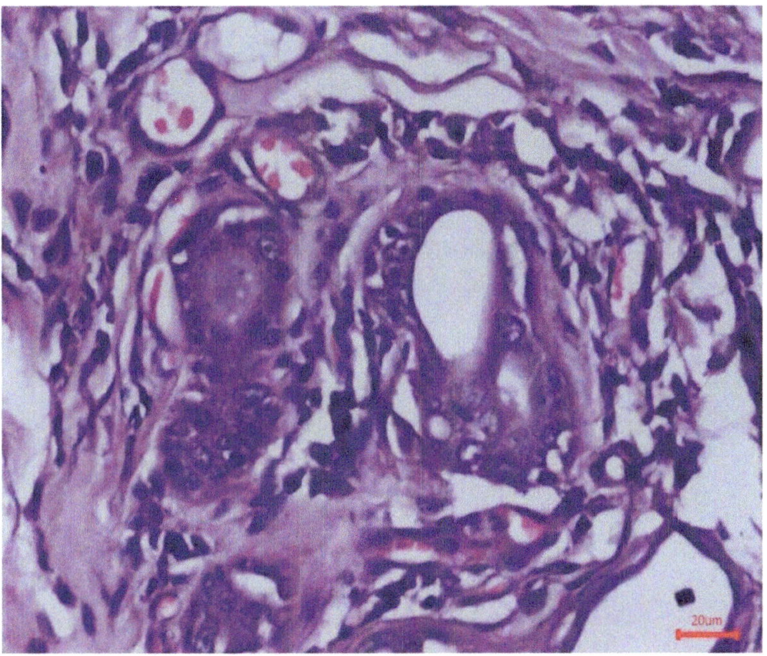

Fig. 20: Sweat gland hyperplasia - Increased number of sweat gland epithelial cells H&E Bar=20 μm

12

Demodicosis (Demodectic Mange/ Demodectic Acariasis)

Etiology

Demodecosis is caused by Demodex species follicular mite with increased numbers. But, it is generally caused by *Demodex canis*. It is divided into two forms – juvenile and adult forms. The juvenile form is more common. This condition may be localized or generalized in nature.

Skin scraping reveals the presence of various stages of demodex mites (Figure 21).

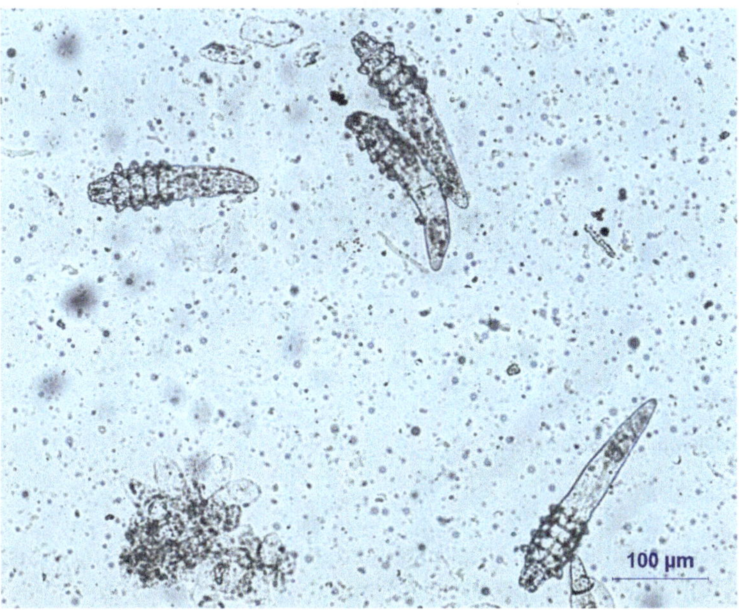

Fig. 21: Skin scraping – Demodecosis - Presence of Demodex mites Bar=100 µm

Gross pathology

The gross lesions manifest itself in two forms: Localised and generalised. Localized demodicosis reveals moderate well demarcated partially alopecic macules, subtle plaques and occasional nodules, erythema, follicular plucking and comedo formation. It is mostly seen in periorbital region, lateral commissures of the mouth, face and forelegs. It is also recorded in bilateral ceruminous otitis externa.

Generalised demodicosis is characterized by multifocal erythematous plaques (Figure 22).

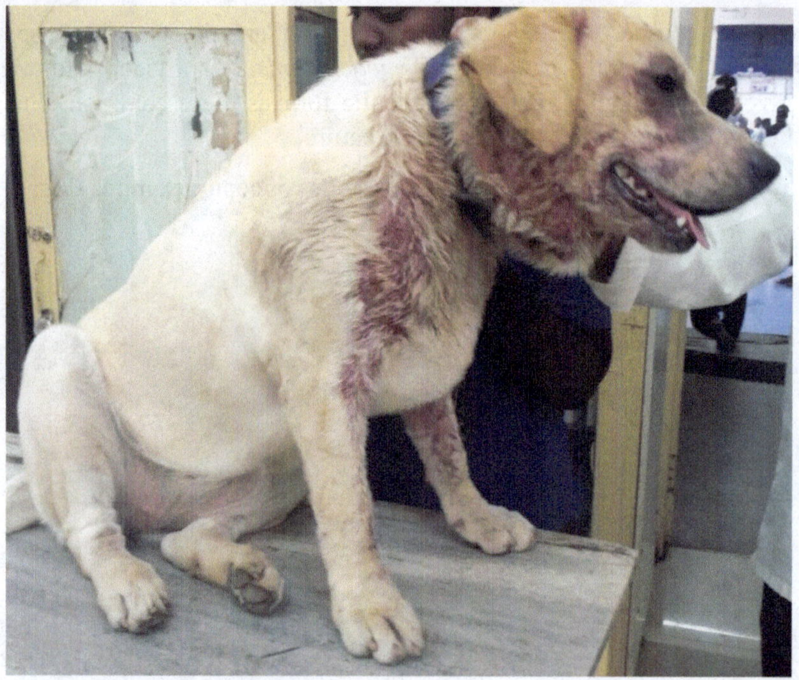

Fig. 22: Demodicosis - Erythematous plaques

Histopathology

Microscopically, epidermis reveals acanthosis, crust and ulceration. Folliculitis, furunculosis, parafollicular granuloma and mural folliculitis are also seen. Variable eosinophilic infiltration is seen. The dilated follicles contain various stages of demodex mites (Figures 23 & 24) surrounded by scanty perifolliculitis and in some cases, demodex mites are present within the large pyogranuloma.

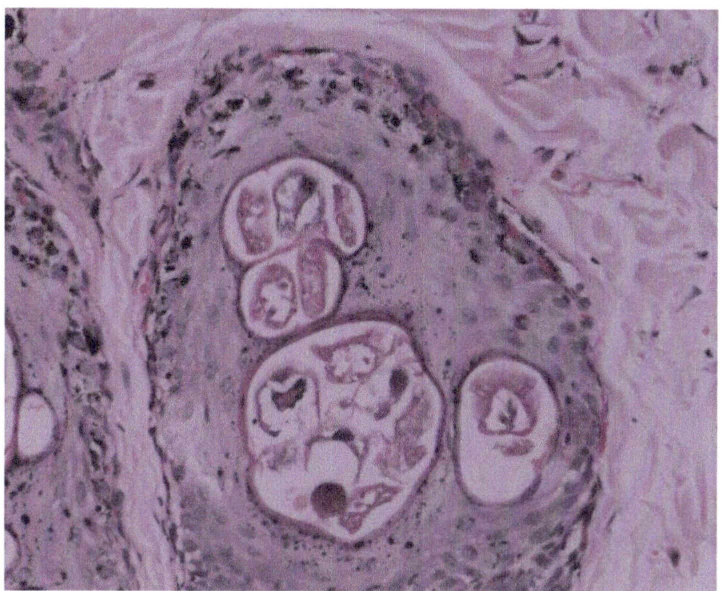

Fig. 23: Demodecosis - Dilated follicle containing various stages of Demodex mites H&E Bar=20μm

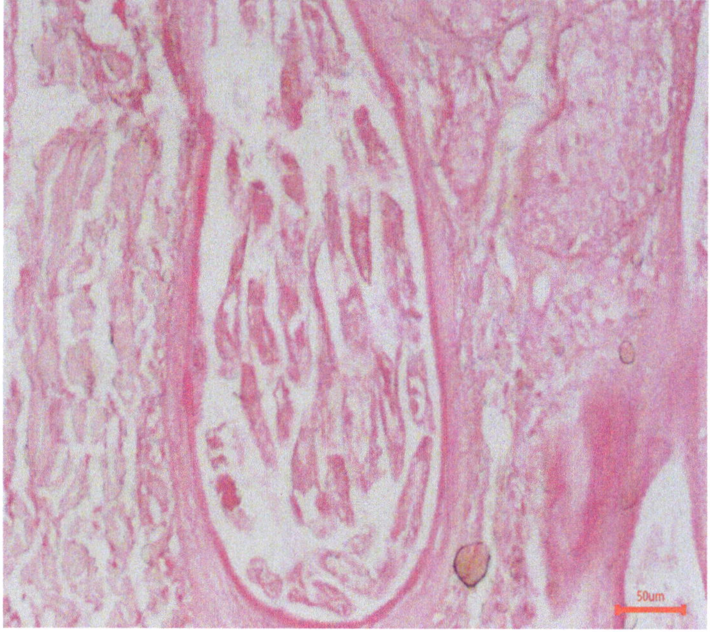

Fig. 24: Demodecosis - Dilated follicle containing various stages of Demodex mites H&E Bar=50 μm

13

Crust

Crust is characterized by the presence of desquamated squamous epithelial cells. The dried exudate consists of necrotic cell debris, leucocytes, RBC's, plasma proteins and microorganisms. It is classified into serous crust (eosinophilic protein exudates), hemorrhagic crust (RBC's), cellular crust (degenerative leucocytes mainly neutrophils), serocellular crust (mixture of serum or plasma or leucocytes) and palisadic crust (presence of leucocytic infiltration, pustules and parakeratosis organized in a horizontal manner).

Histopathology

Microscopically, basophilic debris above the epidermis consisting of degenerative leucocytic nuclei is observed. In hyperkeratosis area, horizontal and vertical palisadic crusts are seen. In Malassezia cases, parakeratotic crust (Figure 25) is seen. In pemphigus cases, acantholytic keratinocytes seen in crust.

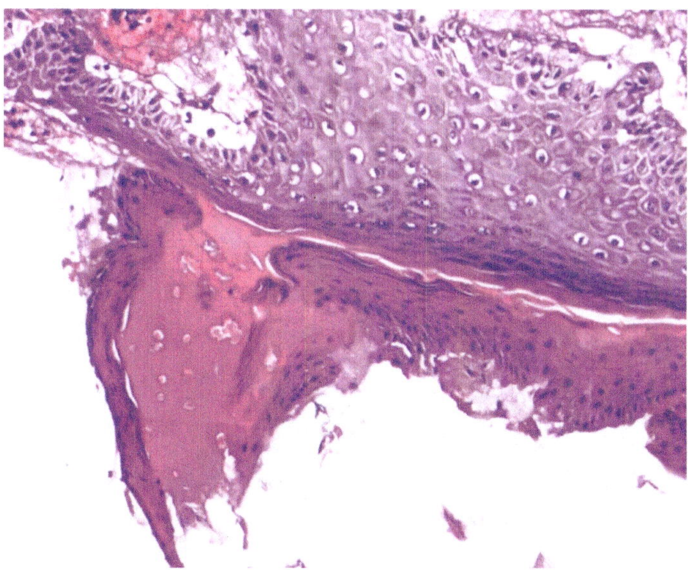

Fig. 25: Presence of parakeratotic crust formation H&E Bar=20μm

14

Scales

Scales are having imperfectly keratinized superficial layers of the epidermis characterized by cracks or thin flakes.

Histopathology

The presence of imperfectly keratinized superficial layers of epidermis and formed as cracks are seen.

15

Ulcers

Ulcerative dermatitis is one of the primary features of the skin disease in which discontinuity of the skin along with marked inflammation and necrosis are seen.

Histopathology

Microscopically, discontinuity of the epidermis and dermis (Figure 26) with necrotic cells and presence of inflammatory cells predominantly degenerative and necrotic neutrophils are seen.

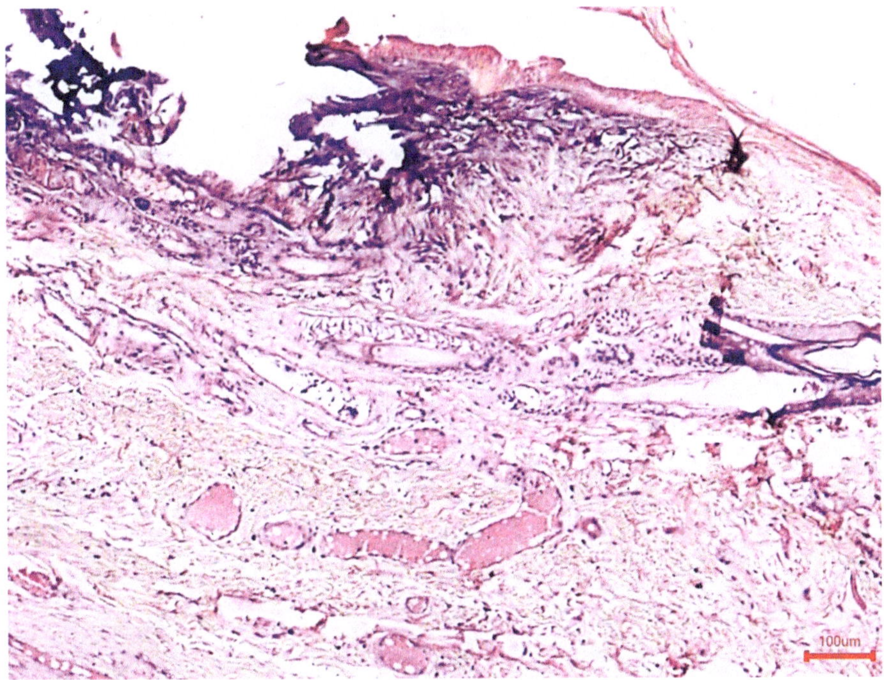

Fig. 26: Ulcer H&E Bar=100 μm

16

Dermatophytosis

Etiology

Canine dermatophytosis (canine ring worm) is a relatively common dermatological condition caused by *Microsporum canis*, *Trichophyton mentagrophytes* and *Microsporum gypseum*. These fungi are keratinophilic in nature. It can occur mostly in the face and forelegs.

Gross pathology

Grossly, erythema, well demarcated and circumscribed alopecic plaques and scales and crust are formed.

Histopathology

Microscopically, acanthosis and hyperkeratosis of epidermis and follicular infundibulum are seen. Dermatophytes can be seen around in protruding hairs or free within the epidermal keratin. It can also produce superficial pustular dermatophytosis (*Trichophyton* spp). Protruding hair shafts are enclosed by keratin and crust. Hair shafts infiltrated and surrounded by dermatophytic dark spores and hyphae.

Presence of perifolliculitis, furunculosis, epidermal hyperplasia, septate hyphae / spores in the hair shaft as well as stratum corneum of epidermis or follicles are seen. Mild to moderate neutrophilic lymphocytic infiltration with macrophages in the follicles is seen.

17

Cheyletiellosis (Cheyletiella dermatitis)

Etiology

It is a pruritic transmissible dermatological condition caused by *Cheyletiella yasguri*, one of the surface living mite.

Gross pathology

Mild scaling, crusting and truncal scaling are seen.

Histopathology

Microscopically, irregular acanthosis and orthokeratotic hyperkeratosis are seen. The keratin layer entrapped with numerous mites in various length are noticed. Perivascular to interstitial infiltration of eosinophils, lymphocytes, macrophages and plasma cells infiltration in the dermis are found.

18

Hair Cycle Disorders of Endocrine Origin

A) Hypothyroidism

Etiology

It is one of the common endocrine disorders of skin of dogs mainly due to deficiency of thyroid hormone followed by cutaneous and non cutaneous signs. It is caused by lymphocytic thyroiditis or idiopathic thyroid necrosis and atrophy. Deficiency of thyroid hormone hinders the metabolic processes throughout the body.

Probable breeds under risk are Chow Chow, Great Dane, Irish Wolfhound, Boxer, Daschund, Doberman Pinscher, Golden Retriever and Irish Setter. But, it may affect any breed. Incidence is recorded in 6 – 10 years of age but any age group may be affected. Neutered dogs are more susceptible to this condition.

Gross pathology

Gross lesions reveal poor hair coat quality, change in coat color, bilateral symmetrical truncal alopecia, alopecia of tail (rat tailed appearance-Figure 27), hyperpigmentation and lichenification.

Other lesions include follicular dysplasia, telogen effluvium, acquired patternalopecia, post clipping alopecia and increased physiological shedding.

Histopathology: Microscopical examination reveals the presence of epidermal and follicular infundibular hyperplasia, variable hyperpigmentation, hairless telogen and thickened follicular infundibulum.

Complete blood count, serum biochemistry and endocrine tests will give confirmatory results.

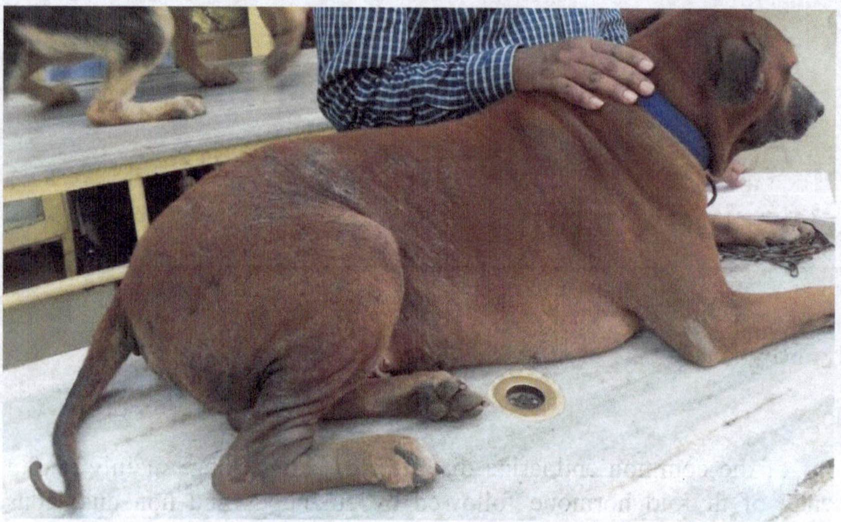

Fig. 27: Hypothyroidism – Dog - Rat tail appearance

Hair cycle disorders of endocrine origin

B) Calcinosis cutis

Etiology

It is a rare dermatological condition with mineral deposition in the dermis, epidermis and subcutis. Usually, it is deposited over the dermal collagen fibers. It may be due to dystrophic calcification accompanied with natural or iatrogenic hyperglucocorticoidism. It is mostly seen in ventral portion of the dog. In non-ulcerated lesion, clinically, chalky white materials with feathery margin are seen.

Gross pathology

Grossly, bilateral symmetrical ulcerated plaques in the ventral part of the abdomen are present (Figure 28). Sometimes, it may change to coalescing erythematous papules (Figure 29). The lesions are firm and gritty.

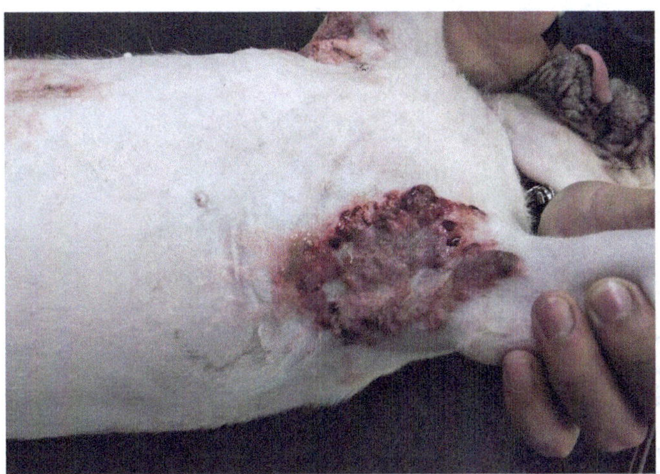

Fig. 28: Calcinosis cutis - Bilateral symmetrical ulcerated plaques in the ventral part of the abdomen

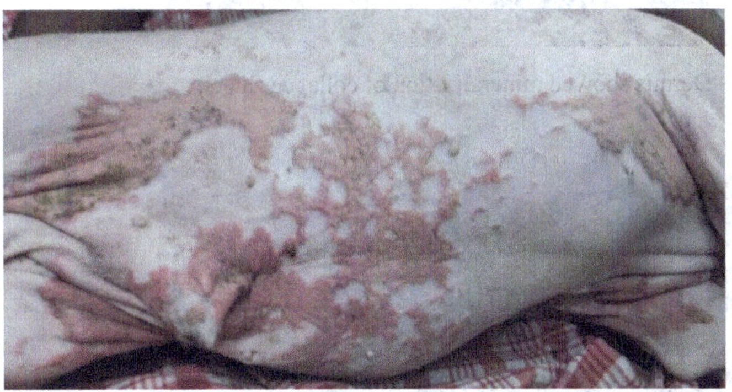

Fig. 29: Calcinosis cutis - Coalescing erythematous papules

Histopathology

Microscopically, it is characterized by the presence of epidermal acanthosis, ulcerated exudates formation and dermal mineralization of collagen fibers (Figure 30). Superficial follicles show hyperplastic changes and infundibular hyperkeratosis. Superficial dermal oedema is also observed. Telogen type atrophy may be present. Dermal collagen of affected areas reveals slightly hypereosinophilic and are severely disrupted. It may be fragmented with deeply basophilic in nature. In early cases, macrophage containing fragmented collagen fibers seen. von kossa stain reveals deposition of dark brown to black mineral materials (Figure 31).

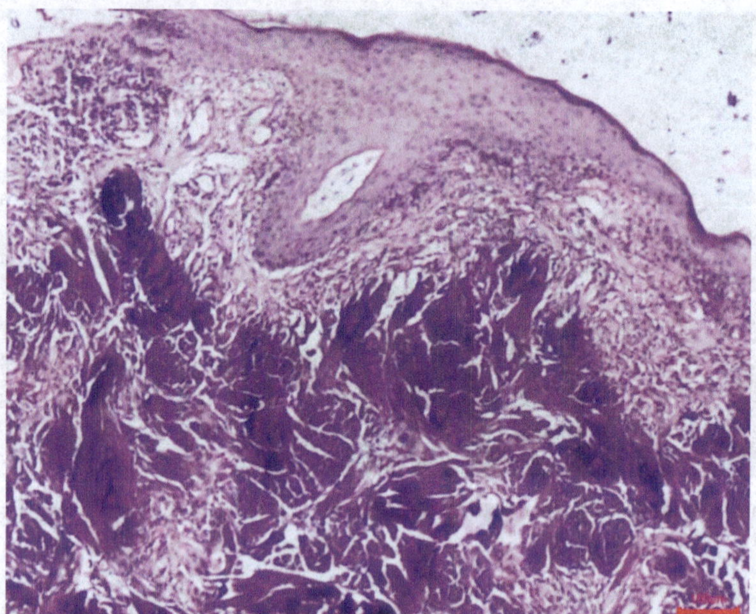

Fig. 30: Calcinosis cutis - Dermis showed mineralization of collagen fibers. H&E Bar=100μm

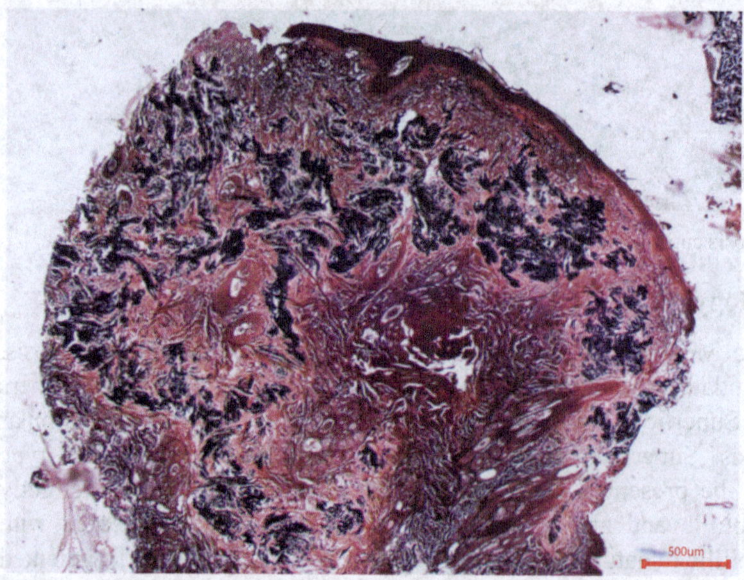

Fig. 31: Calcinosis cutis - Dermis showed dark brown to black coloured mineral deposition of collagen fibres. von kossa Bar=100 μm

Hair cycle disorders of endocrine origin

C) Hyperoestrogenism (Canine Female Hyperoestrogenism)

Etiology

It is one of the rare endocrine associated skin disease arising due to excessive estrogen or imbalance of sex hormone ratio. It is more common in sexually active bitches with cystic ovarian conditions or ovarian tumors. It is also due to excessive administration of estrogen as a therapy for urinary incontinence in spayed dogs.

Gross pathology

Gross lesions reveal bilateral symmetrical alopecia and macular hyperpigmentation in anogenital orifice followed by abdomen, thigh, chest, flank and neck. Lightened coat color and darker hairs are also seen. Mammary gland enlargement (gynaecomastia), nipple enlargement, vulvar enlargement and secondary infections such as Malassezia dermatitis may occur. Naturally occurring cases have been reported in French and English bull dogs.

Histopathology

Microscopically, lesions look like sertoli cell associated skin disease of male dogs. Epidermis and follicular epithelium show acanthosis, hyperpigmentation and hair less telogen follicles. Infiltration of neutrophils and mononuclear cells are also observed.

19

Canine Zinc Responsive Dermatosis

Etiology

It is a rare canine dermatological condition. This condition is subdivided into two groups. In the first group, it is seen in Siberian husky and Alaskan malamutes. It is due to inherited impairment in the zinc absorption or metabolism. In the second group, it is due to use of high plant phytates diet (zinc absorption prevention), commercial or home prepared diet which is zinc deficient or diet is over supplemented with calcium and other vitamins and minerals which impair zinc absorption. Group two is mostly seen in large breed dogs and young adults.

Gross pathology

Externally, the lesions seen in group one includes erythema, thick adherent scales, crust, alopecia and lichenification in mucocutaneous junctions, genital and pressure points. Whereas, in group two, there will be presence of thick well demarcated crusts and lichenified plaques with erosion or ulcers (Figure 32).

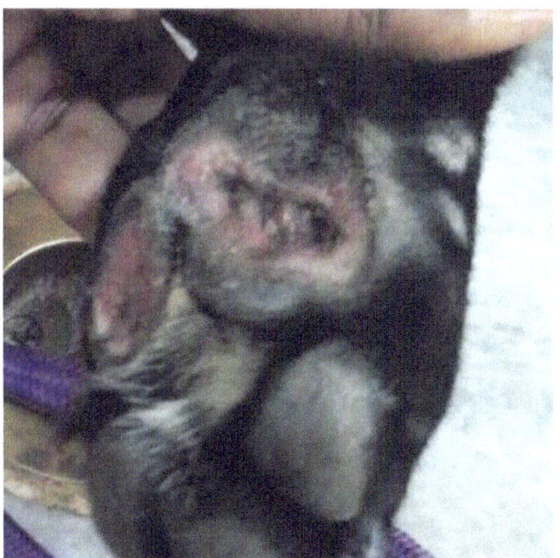

Fig. 32: Zinc dermatosis – Dog - Well demarcated crusts, erosions and ulcers

Histopathology

Microscopically, severe acanthosis, parakeratosis and spongiosis of the epidermis are seen. Dermal neutrophilic and mononuclear cell infiltration is also present. In between the parakeratotic layer, serum is also present.

20

Acanthosis Nigricans

Etiology

It is a rare idiopathic primary dermatitis condition seen mainly in Daschund.

Gross pathology

It is characterized by presence of bilaterally symmetrical axillary hyperpigmentation, lichenification and alopecia. In severe cases, greasy odoriferous keratinous debris accumulations are seen. It is mostly seen in the axilla and groin region.

Histopathology

Microscopically, there is a mild to moderate acanthosis (Figure 33), hyperkeratosis, focal parakeratosis and follicular keratosis. Basal layer keratinocytes are mostly hyperpigmented. The dermis reveals mild to moderate superficial perivascular interstitial lymphocytes, macrophages, a few plasma cells and neutrophils. Continuous production of the pigments in the basal cell keratinocytes is seen.

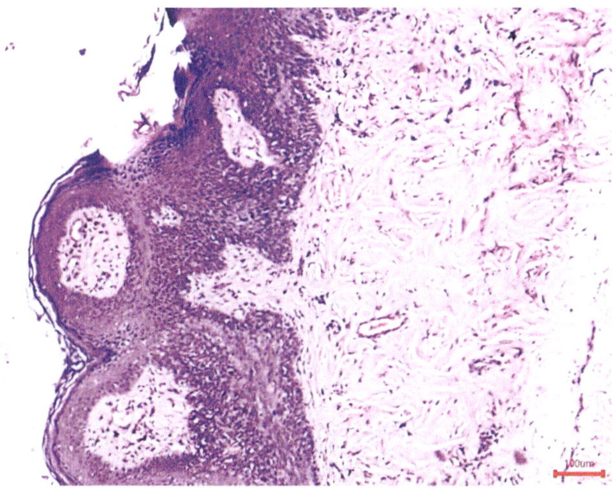

Fig. 33: Dog - Acanthosis and mild perivascular mononuclear cell infiltration H&E Bar=100

21

Eosinophilic Granuloma (Canine Collagenolytic Granuloma)

Etiology

It is a relatively rare skin disease or dermatologic condition. Hypersensitivity reaction is one of the suggestive cause for this condition characterized by nodules or plaques which are seen in the skin, oral mucosa and external ear canal. Hypersensitivity accompanied with eosinophilia in tissue and blood is seen. Eosinophilic degranulation is also observed.

Gross pathology

Gross lesions include the presence of papules, nodules, plaques and ulcers in the skin. Arthropod infestation may also stimulate mouth eosinophilic granuloma.

Histopathology

Microscopically, the epidermis reveals acanthosis, necrosis, ulcer, superficial to deep perivascular to diffuse infiltration of eosinophils (Figure 34) along with oedema and mucin. Eosinophilic degranulation is seen around the individual collagen fibers to form flame figures. Granuloma is arranged in palisadic pattern along with collagen fibers. The flame figures have peripheral radiating projection surrounded by eosinophils, macrophage and a few giant cells to form granuloma. Oral eosinophilic granuloma is characterized by the presence of eosinophils, flame figures and macrophage and multinucleated giant cells.

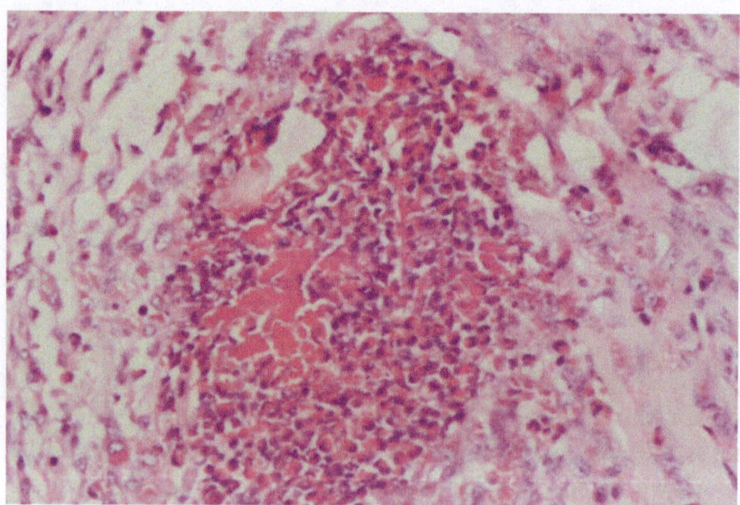

Fig. 34: Canine eosinophilic granuloma - Perivascular to diffuse infiltration of eosinophils H&E Bar=20μm

22

Sertoli Cell Tumor Associated Skin Disease

Etiology

It is an uncommon endocrine related skin disorder. It is very rarely encountered in neutered dogs. It is always associated with cryptorchidism and sertoli cell tumor. This condition is closely accompanied with endocrine related testicular tumor followed by skin lesion and feminization.

Gross pathology

Gross lesions are characterised by bilateral symmetrical alopecia in the perineum and genital followed by abdomen, chest, flank and neck. Coat colour is lighter with black or dark brown hairs. Focal macular melanosis, lichenification and alopecia are also observed. In gynaecomastia, nipple enlargement and pendulous nipples with galactorrhoea are seen. Well demarcated, linear band of macular erythema and mottled hyperpigmentation or comedones on the ventral prepuce of dogs are characteristic cutaneous marker of male feminizing syndrome.

Histopathology

Microscopical examination shows acanthosis, follicular infundibular hyperplasia and increased melanin pigmentation in the epidermis. Follicular atrophy and hairless telogen follicles are seen in more numbers.

23

Malassezia Dermatitis

A very common condition caused by Malassezia pachydermatis in dogs. It is also caused by predisposing allergic skin disease. It occurs in ventral neck, ventral abdomen, axilla, face, pinnae, feet and forelegs. Tape impression smear will reveal numerous yeasts.

Gross pathology

Gross findings reveal presence of erythema, greasy to waxy scales, crust and alopecia, lichenification and hyperpigmentation (Figure 35).

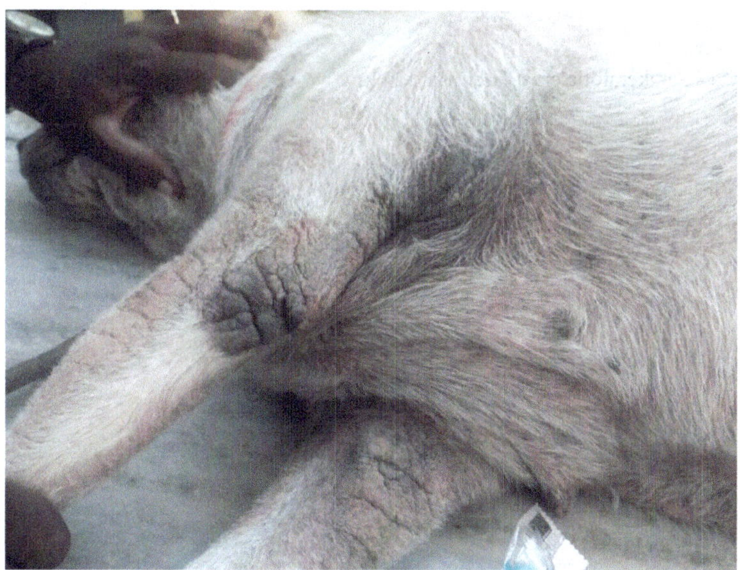

Fig. 35: Malassezia – Dog - Lichenification and alopecia

Histopathology

Microscopically, acanthosis, spongiosis, hyperkeratosis, parakeratotic crusts (Figure 36) and presence of yeasts in the keratin are seen (Figure 37).

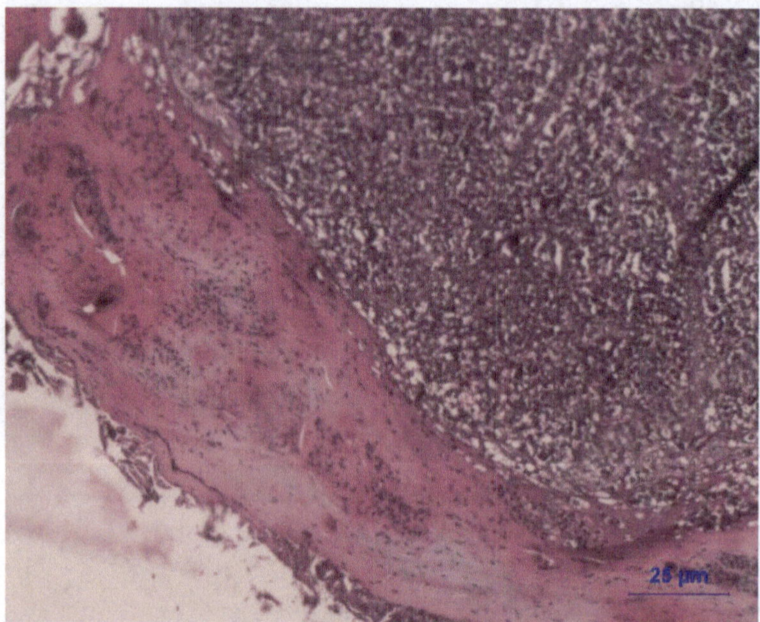

Fig. 36: Malassezia - Parakeratotic crust H&E Bar=25 µm

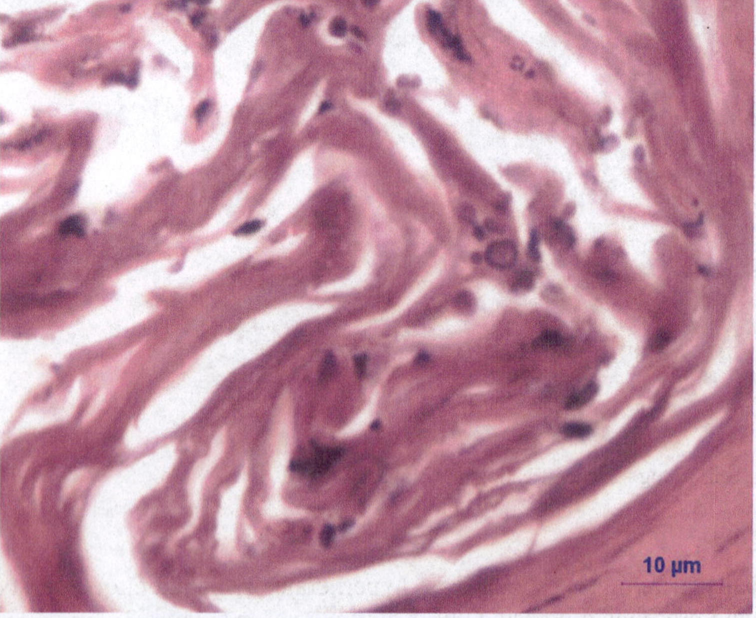

Fig. 37: Malassezia - Presence of yeasts in the keratin H&E Bar=10µm

Cutaneous Neoplasm – Epithelial Tumors

24

Papilloma

It is a benign tumor of squamous epithelial cells. Papilloma may be caused by virus in dogs. Papillomas usually vary in size measuring about 0.5 to 6 mm..

Grossly, the lesions are usually pedunculated (Figure 38) and solitary. It is mostly seen on the face, eyelid, feet, conjunctiva etc.

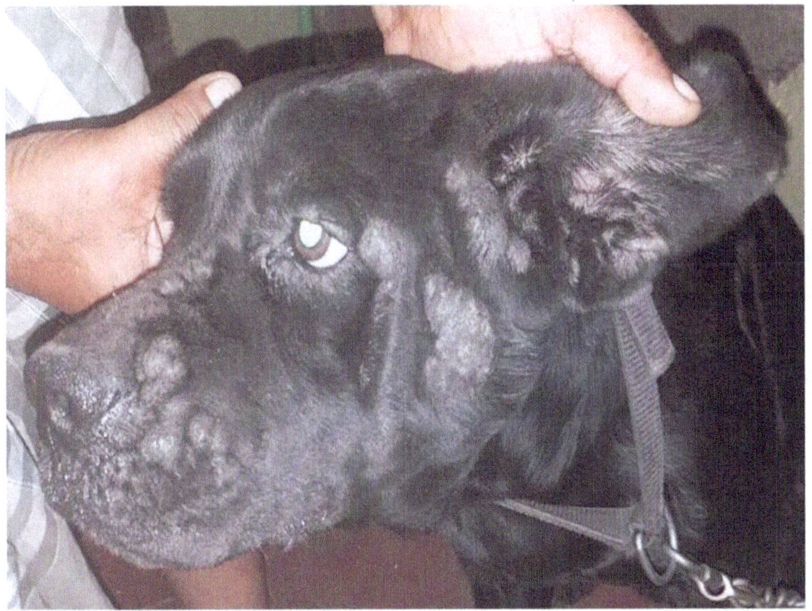

Fig. 38: Papilloma - Pedunculated and cauliflower like growth

Cytologically, numerous mature squamous epithelial cells and prominent round to variable sized nuclei with basophilic cytoplasm are seen.

Histologically, elongated dermal papillae with acanthotic parakeratotic epidermis, finger-like projections (Figure 39) and mild inflammation will be seen. Papillated cytoplasm in the stratum spinosum is observed.

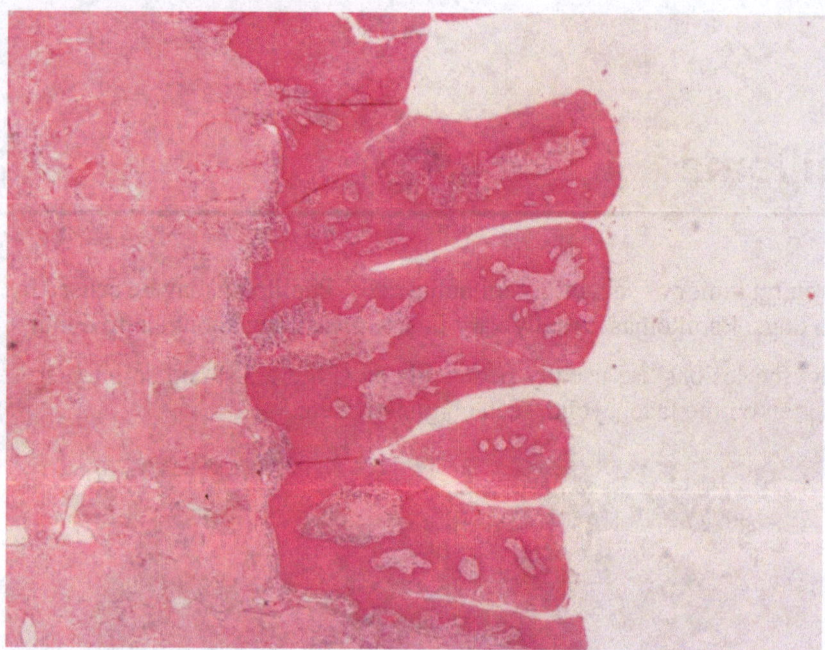

Fig. 39: Papilloma - Elongated dermal papillae with acanthosis, finger- like projections fibrovascular core H&E 4x

25

Squamous Cell Carcinoma

This tumour may occur due to specific mutation in the p53 tumor suppressor gene. This is one of the most common epithelial tumor of dog. It is classified into well differentiated, moderately differentiated and poorly differentiated tumour.

Grossly, papillary-like growth or cauliflower-like growth measuring about a few mm to several cm may be visualized. It may be single (Figure 40) or multiple. In some of the cases, it may be crateriform. It is mostly seen in ventral abdomen and medial stifle region.

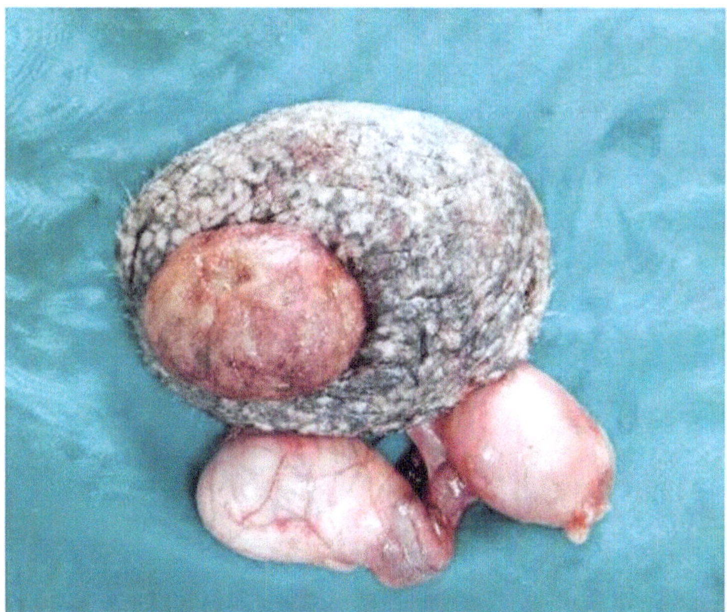

Fig. 40: Squamous cell carcinoma - Scrotal skin - Single nodule

Cytologically, clusters of neoplastic squamous cells of small to medium sized round to squamous cells with very basophilic cytoplasm, large round nuclei, coarse chromatin and multiple prominent nucleoli are seen. Tadpole appearance of the cells is also seen.

Histopathologically, well differentiated squamous cell carcinoma appears like islands of neoplastic polyhedral shaped squamous cells with numerous keratin pearls (Figure 41) and neutrophilic infiltration with abundant fibrovascular connective tissue also observed. Cytoplasm is amphophilic, nuclei large and vesicular. Mitotic figures are moderately low. Moderately differentiated squamous cell carcinoma shows presence of islands of neoplastic squamous cells with a few to moderate number of keratin pearls. Cells are polyhedral shaped containing amphophilic cytoplasm and vesicular nuclei with multiple prominent nucleoli. The neoplastic cells are arranged in cords or nests or islands. In poorly differentiated squamous cell carcinoma, keratin pearls are absent or few. The cells show amphophilic cytoplasm containing hyperchromatic nuclei with prominent multiple nucleoli and moderate to high mitotic figures. It is of anaplastic type. Immunohistochemical detection of squamous cell carcinoma can be done by using Cytokeratin AE1/AE3 which shows positivity in the cytoplasm.

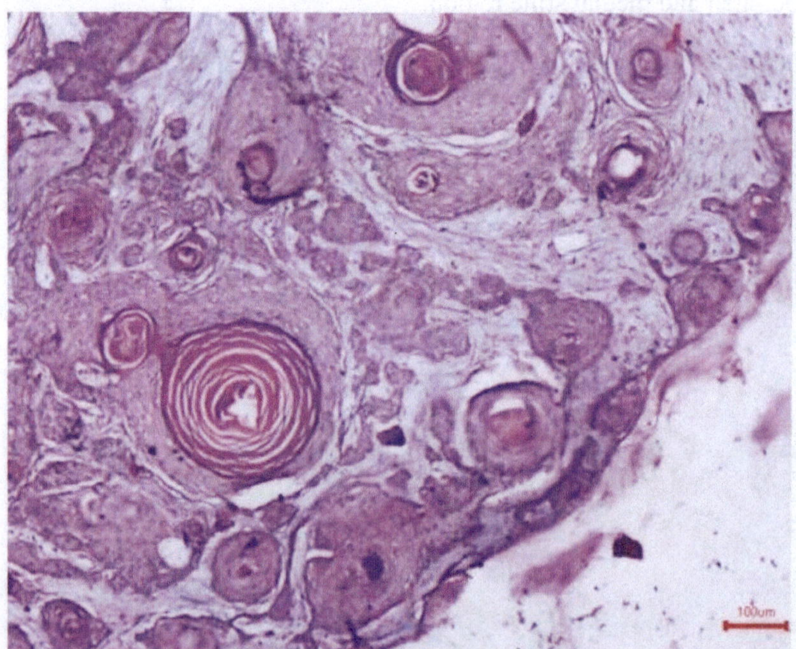

Fig. 41: Squamous cell carcinoma - Note keratin pearls H&E Bar=100 μm

26

Basal Cell Carcinoma (Trichoblastoma)

Basal cell carcinoma is a locally malignant epithelial tumor of skin which is mainly composed of basal cells. This may occur due to mutation in the tumor suppressor gene p53 and chronic exposure to UV radiation.

Cytologically, neoplastic cylindrical columnar cells, are moderate to high in number. The neoplastic cells are small to medium sized with round to spherical nuclei with basophilic cytoplasm (Figure 42 & 43).

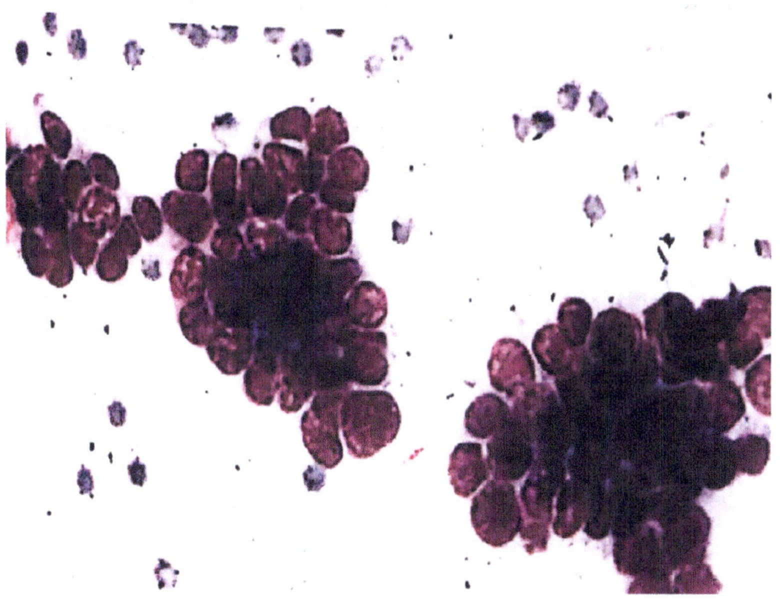

Fig. 42: Basal Cell carcinoma – Cytology – Clusters of tightly adherent cells with oval nucleiand sparse cytoplasm WG 800x (Image Courtesy: Krithiga *et al.*, 2005)

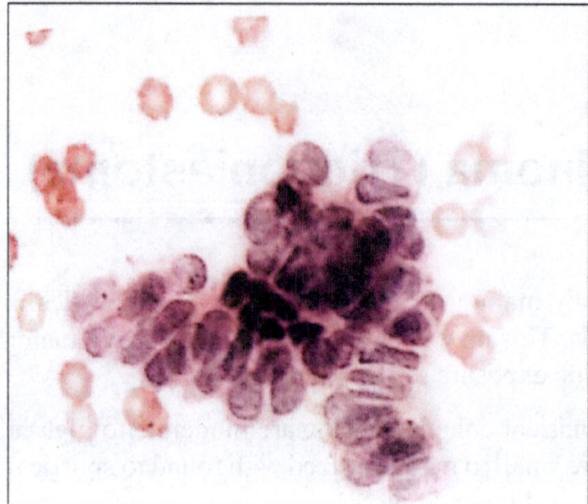

Fig. 43: Basal Cell carcinoma – Cytology – Tightly adherent cuboidal cells with oval nuclei H&E 1000x (*Courtesy*: Krithiga et al., 2005)

Grossly, ulcerated, or poorly to well circumscribed, pink to grey white colored mass is mostly present in the head, fore head (Figure 44), neck and base of ear. Cut section of the cases show multilobulated pattern. The size of the mass ranges from 0.5 to 18 cm.

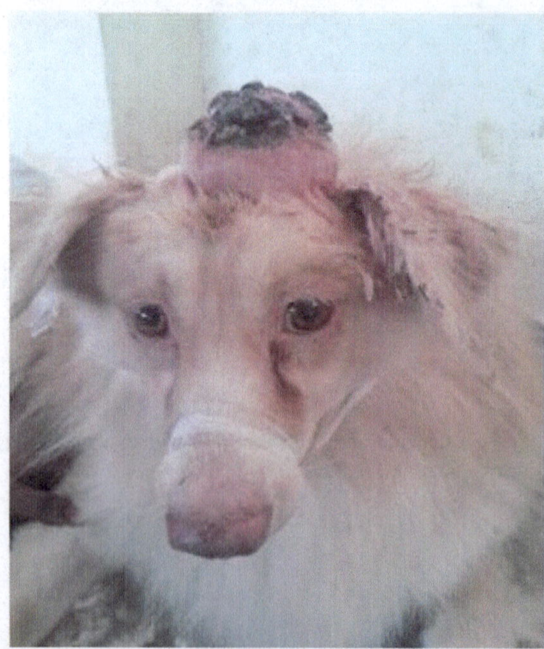

Fig. 44: Basal Cell Carcinoma – Forehead

Histopathologically, basal cell carcinoma reveals the following patterns of solid, ribbon (Figure 45 & 46), medusoid, adenoid and cystic. Some cases show baso-squamous cell type. In ribbon type, cells are in palisading appearance with prominent nucleoli and small amount of cytoplasm. Hyperchromatic nuclei with inconspicuous nucleoli and mitotic figures variable in number are noticed.

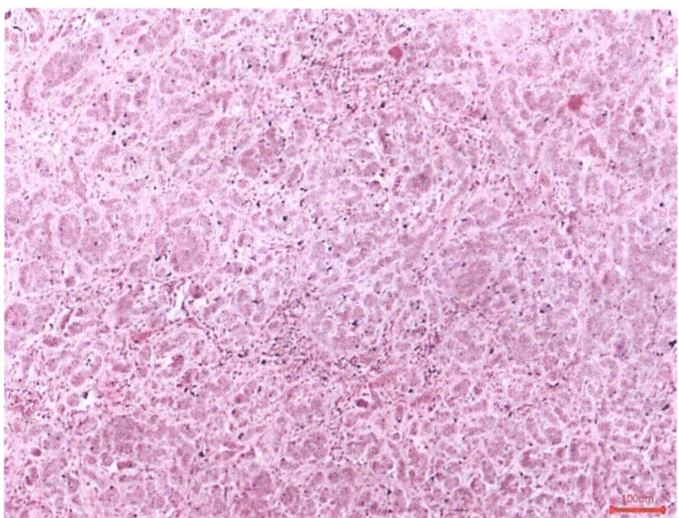

Fig. 45: Basal Cell Carcinoma - Ribbon type H&E Bar=100 μm

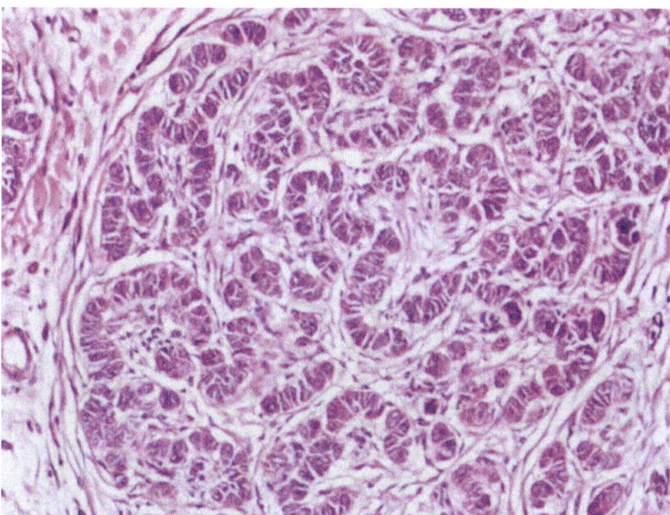

Fig. 46: Basal Cell Carcinoma - Ribbon and serpent type H&E 20x

27

Sweat Gland Adenoma and Adenocarcinoma

This is a benign/malignant tumor originating from the apocrine and eccrine sweat glands in dogs. It is usually recorded in the head and neck region but it may occur on any site.

Cytology reveals clusters of moderate to severe exfoliated neoplastic cells which contain round nuclei slightly eccentric in position in the light pale granular cytoplasm. In carcinomas, clusters of basophilic epithelial cells had large nuclei and prominent nucleoli. It may also contain one or two large secretory droplets.

Grossly, these tumors are mostly solitary type and circumscribed soft to firm elevated tumors (Figure 47) and they are often ulcerated. Ulcerated forms are mostly seen in carcinomas.

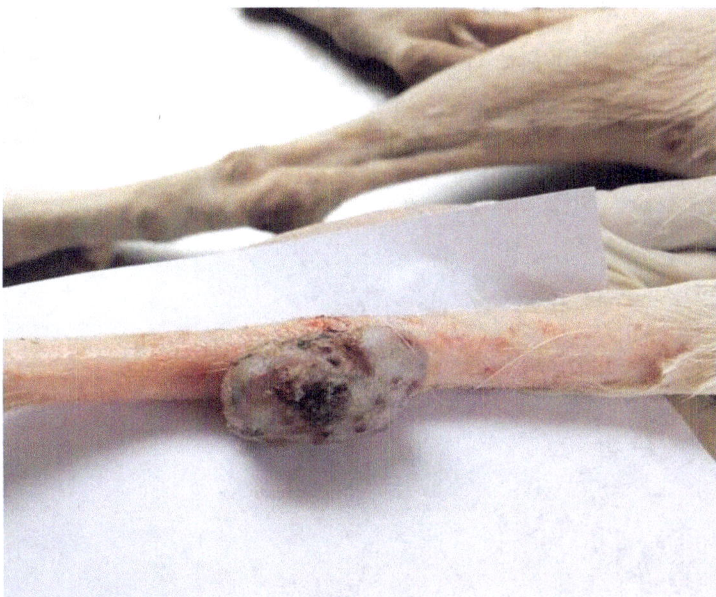

Fig. 47: Sweat gland adenoma of tail – Solitary

Microscopical examination reveals cystic, glandular and ductular (Figure 48) adenoma. Adenomas lined by single cuboidal to columnar epithelial layer, have abundant granular eosinophilic cytoplasm and basally placed small nuclei. Carcinomas are mostly arranged in various types ranging from solitary, tubulopapillary, glandular, ductular to clear and signet ring shape. In carcinomas, majority of neoplastic cells have round to oval hyperchromatic nuclei with prominent nucleoli and also contain abundant eosinophilic cytoplasm with indistinct cell borders (Figure 49). Mitotic figures are also observed in variable numbers.

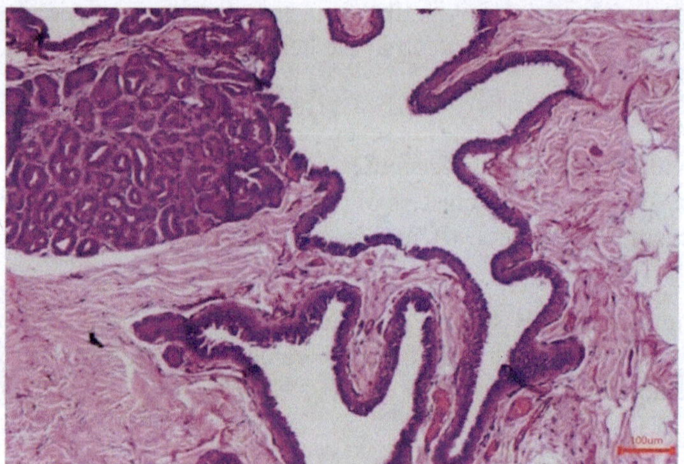

Fig. 48: Sweat gland adenoma H&E Bar=100 μm

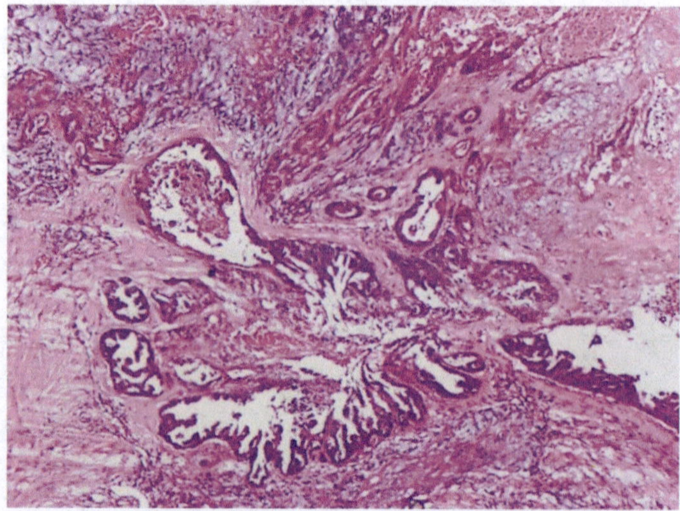

Fig. 49: Sweat gland adenocarcinoma – Papillary pattern H&E 4x

28

Sebaceous Gland Adenoma and Adenocarcinoma

It is one of the common epithelial skin tumors. It is more common in head but also recorded in other sites such as back, tail, limb, trunk and eyelids. It is a tumor of sebaceous cells. In sebaceous gland adenoma, it has predominantly sebocytes with less of basaloid reserve cells while in sebaceous epithelioma variant, more of basaloid reserve cells are seen with less of sebocytes.

Grossly, the tumor shows elevated multiple nodular masses associated with alopecia, hyperpigmentation and ulceration. The color is pale yellow to white. It may be multilobulated by connective tissue trabecular division.

Cytologically, adenoma shows clusters of basal cells which have round to ovoid centrally placed nuclei with moderate clear to foamy cytoplasm. Carcinomas have group of pleomorphic basal cells with anisokaryosis, altered nuclear cytoplasmic ratio and mitotic figures.

Histopathologically, the tumors reveal multilobules separated by connective tissue trabeculae (Figure 50). Periphery of the lobule reveals small basophilic reserve cells with hyperchromatic nuclei and scanty cytoplasm. Mitotic figures are scanty in number. In carcinomas, neoplastic cells have multilobulated appearance separated by connective tissue trabeculae and variable sized intracytoplasmic lipid vacuoles (Figure 51). Nucleus of the neoplastic cells is medium to large hyperchromatic nuclei with prominent nucleoli. Mitotic figures are seen in variable numbers.

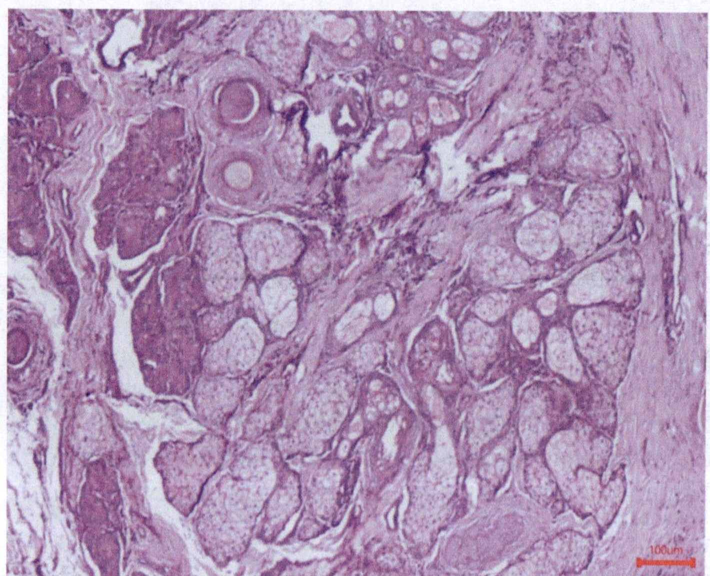

Fig. 50: Sebaceous gland adenoma – Multiple lobules separated by connective tissue trabeculae H&E Bar = 100 µm

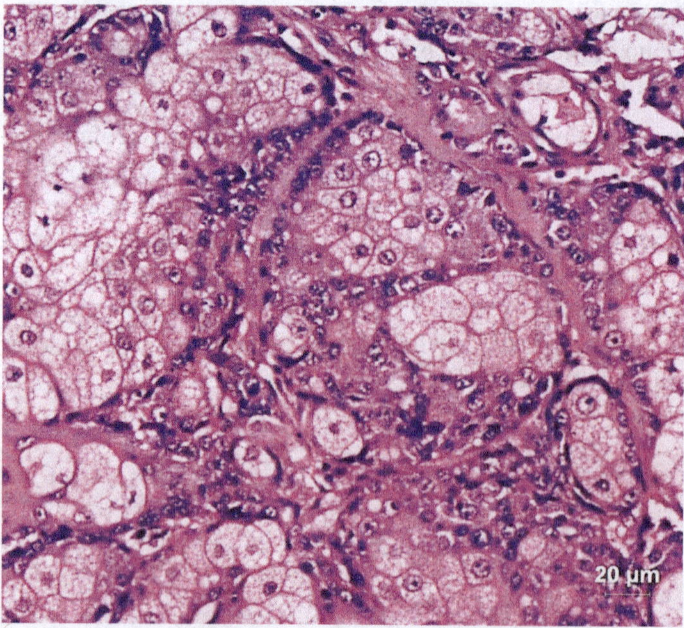

Fig. 51: Sebaceous gland adenocarcinoma – Multilobulated and variable sized intracytoplasmic vacuoles H&E Bar = 20 µm

29

Ceruminous Gland Adenoma and Adenocarcinoma

The tumor arising out of ceruminous gland might develop subsequent to chronic otitis externa in dogs. It may be a benign or malignant tumor of ceruminous gland epithelium. It is more common in the external ear canal of dogs.

Cytology reveals numerous clusters of round cells with hyperchromatic eccentrically placed nuclei in the moderate cytoplasm and anisocytosis.

Grossly, mostly single to multiple nodules (Figure 52) are seen in the ear canal particularly in the vertical ear canal. These appear as gray white to dark brown colored mass when they get inspissated for a long period of time.

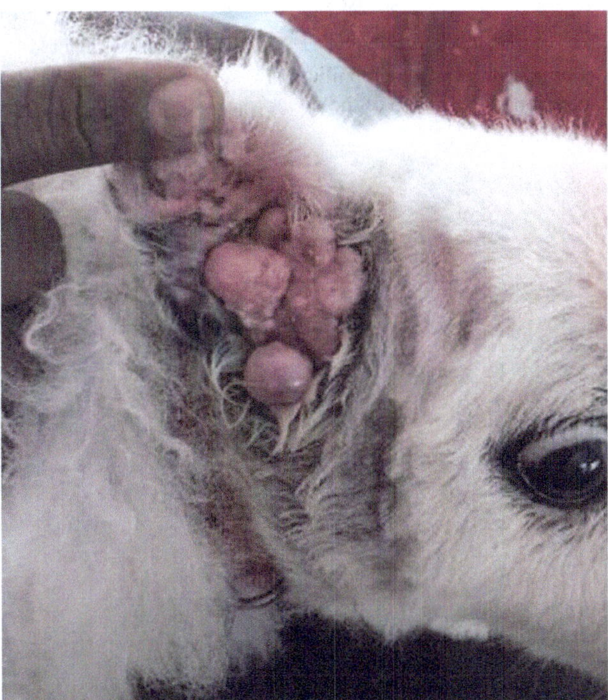

Fig. 52: Multiple gray white nodules

Microscopically, in the benign type, ceruminous gland tumor shows brown material retention in the glandular lumen (Figure 53) and small brown globules within the cytoplasm of the neoplastic cells. In carcinoma, these are infiltrative and erosive, ulcerated with the presence of large prominent nuclei with large nucleoli. Cytoplasm contains abundant eosinophilic cytoplasm. Copper coloured secretion is usually present in the lumen of the acini and duct (Figure 54). Mitotic figures are commonly seen.

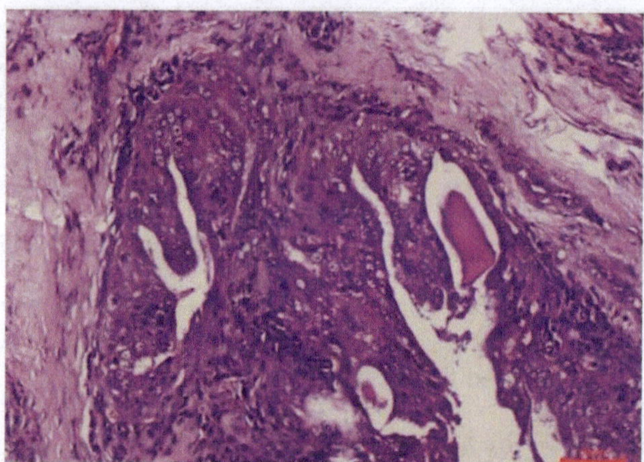

Fig. 53: Ceruminous gland adenoma-Abundant eosinophilic cytoplasm with copper colored secretion in the lumen of the acini and duct H&E Bar = 100 μm

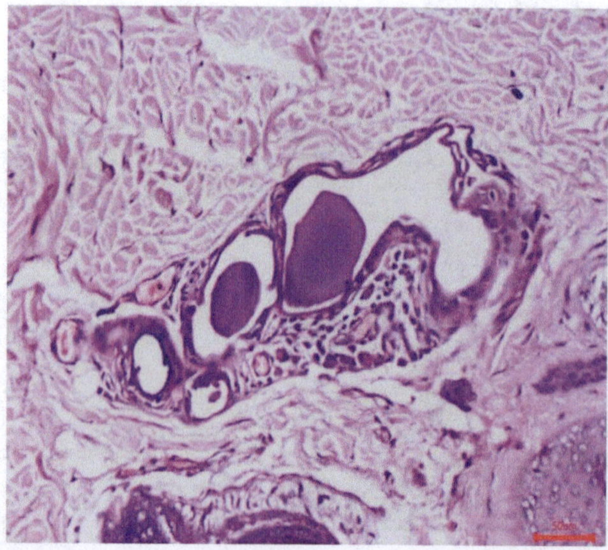

Fig. 54: Ceruminous gland adenoma- Brown material retention in the glandular lumen H&E Bar=50 μm

30

Perianal Gland Adenoma and Adenocarcinoma

Perianal gland tumors originate around the anus of the dog, upper and lower part of the tail and prepucial area. Retention of gonadal hormone receptors is one of the causes for perianal gland adenoma and adenocarcinoma.

Cytology reveals the presence of hepatoid cells with centrally placed nuclei and prominent nucleoli. A small flattened reserve cells or resting cells are also noticed around the hepatoid cells. In malignant variety, the cells containing large vesicular nuclei, eosinophilic granular cytoplasm and binucleated cells, mitotic figures, reserve cells, moderate stroma and lymphoplasmacytic infiltration are seen (Figure 55 & 56).

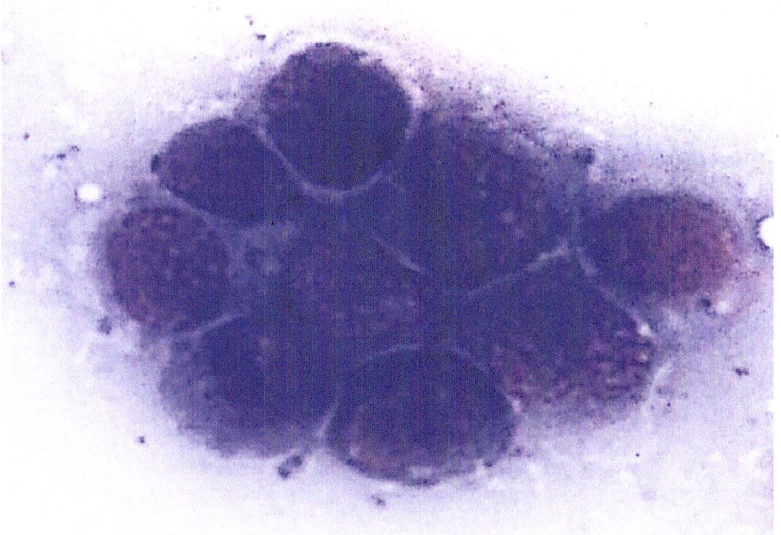

Fig. 55: Perianal gland adenoma – Hepatoid cell clusters with spherical nucleus and granular chromatin WG 1000x (Image Courtesy - Krithiga et al., 2005)

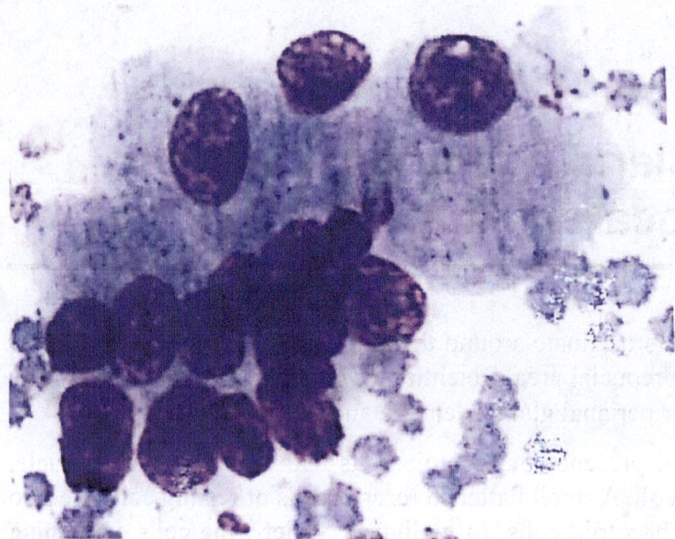

Fig. 56: Cluster of hepatoid cells with granular cytoplasm. Note reserve cells. WG 1000x (Image courtesy – Krithiga et al., 2005)

Grossly, these are solitary in type (Figure 57) to multiple nodules. The size ranges from 1cm to more than 10 cm. It may be ulcerated and haemorrhagic in nature.

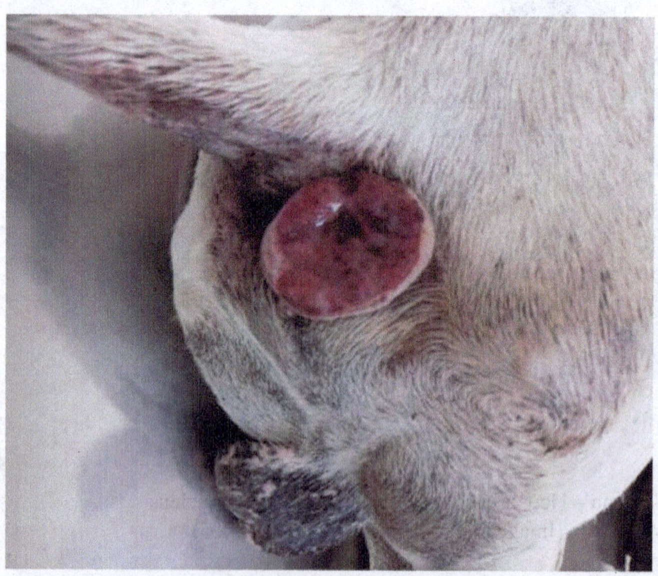

Fig. 57: Perianal gland adenocarcinoma – Solitary mass of 4 cm in diameter around the perianal region

Histopathologically, adenoma reveals round to polyhedral shaped cells with centrally placed large ovoid vesicular nuclei with prominent small nucleoli and abundant cytoplasm (Figure 58). Mitotic figures are observed. It is seen surrounding the reserve cells. In carcinomas, they show disorderly growth containing large polyhedral cells and reserve cells (Figure 59) without lobulation. Anisokaryosis, anisocytosis and mitotic figures are seen. Squamous metaplasia is also seen. Tumor cell invasion into the adjacent connective tissue and lymphatic tissue is observed.

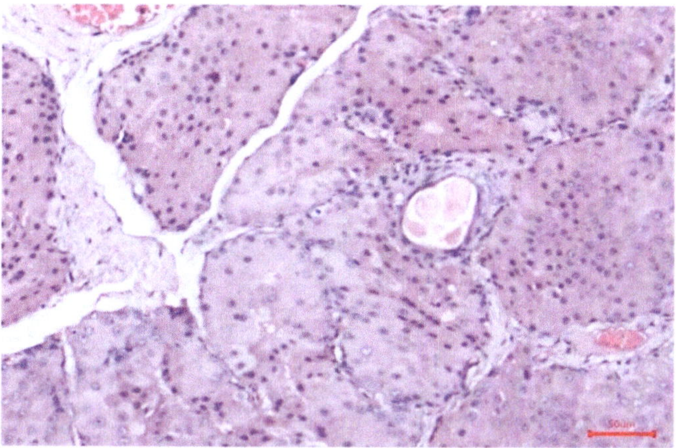

Fig. 58: Perianal adenoma – Round to polyhedral shaped cells with centrally placed large ovoid vesicular nuclei with abundant cytoplasm H&E Bar = 50 μm

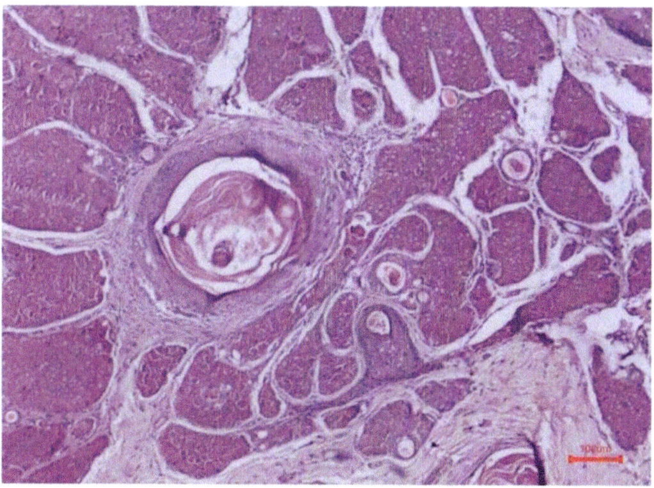

Fig. 59: Perianal adenocarcinoma – Disorderly growth containing large polyhedral cells and reserve cells H&E Bar = 100 μm

31

Fibroma

Benign/malignant tumor may arise from fibrous tissue. Fibroma mostly occurs in the dermis or subcutis of limbs and head.

Gross pathology

Grossly, the tumour occurs mostly as round, soft, firm (Figure 60) rubbery round or oval and dome shape. These may also be pedunculated and grey white on cut section. Some of them are ulcerated and haemorrhagic.

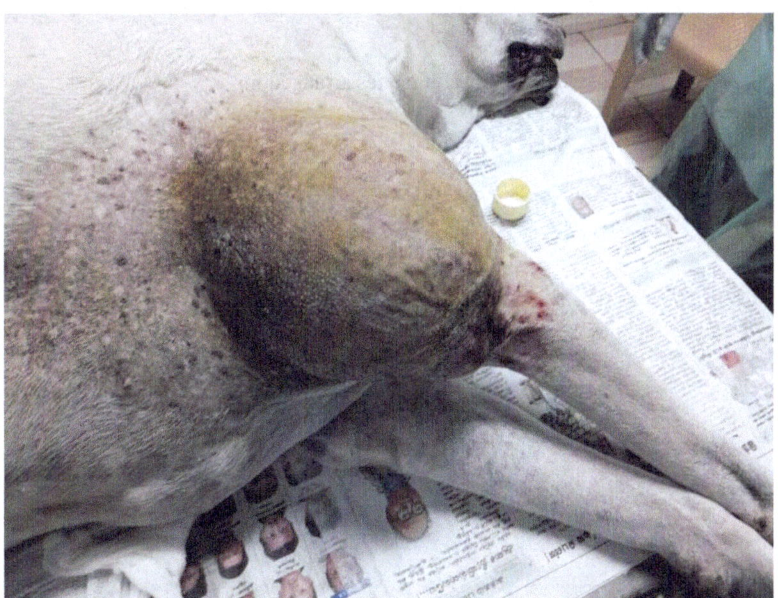

Fig. 60: Fibroma - Elbow joint - Round soft firm nodule

Cytology reveals individual uniform sized spindle shaped cells with moderate amount of light blue cytoplasm and round to ovoid nuclei with one or two small indistinct nucleoli.

Histopathologically, well circumscribed mature fibrocytes are arranged in interlacing bundles (Figure 61) and are rarely in whorl pattern. Indistinct cytoplasm with scanty to absent mitotic figures are seen.

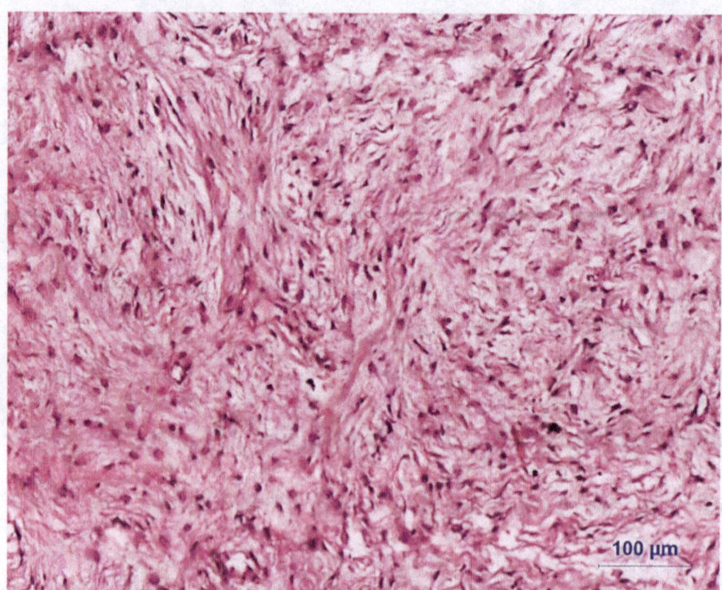

Fig. 61: Fibroma - Well circumscribed mature fibrocytes arranged in interlacing bundles pattern H&E Bar=100 µm

32

Fibrosarcoma

The tumour is most commonly seen in adult and aged dogs. It occurs anywhere on the body surface. It is due to trauma, chronic inflammation, vaccination, genetic predisposition etc.

Grossly, well circumscribed (Figure 62) to infiltrative type with no encapsulation. The cut surface is grey white and glistening. Interwoven fascicular pattern is also often seen.

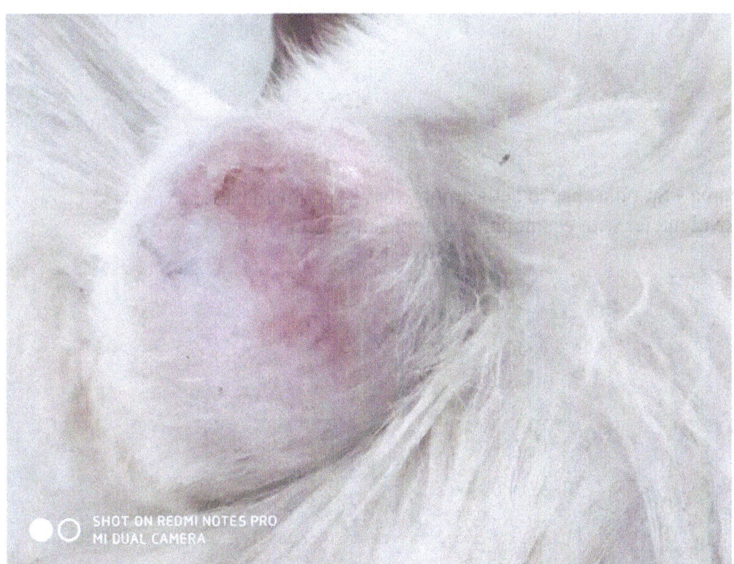

Fig. 62: Fibrosarcoma - Above right elbow joint - Well circumscribed

Cytologically, fibrosarcoma reveals the presence of plump to oval cells with indistinct cytoplasm, altered nuclear to cytoplasmic ratio, prominent angular nucleoli and multinucleated cells.

Histopathologically, the tumour consists of presence of well differentiated spindle shaped neoplastic cells (Figure 63) arranged in interwoven or herringbone pattern, elongated to oval nuclei with inconspicuous nucleoli with scanty cytoplasm. The anaplastic type shows more pleomorphism. Mitotic figures are varied in number.

Immunohistochemistry by using vimentin reveals strong expression of brown coloured reaction in the cytoplasm (Figure 64)

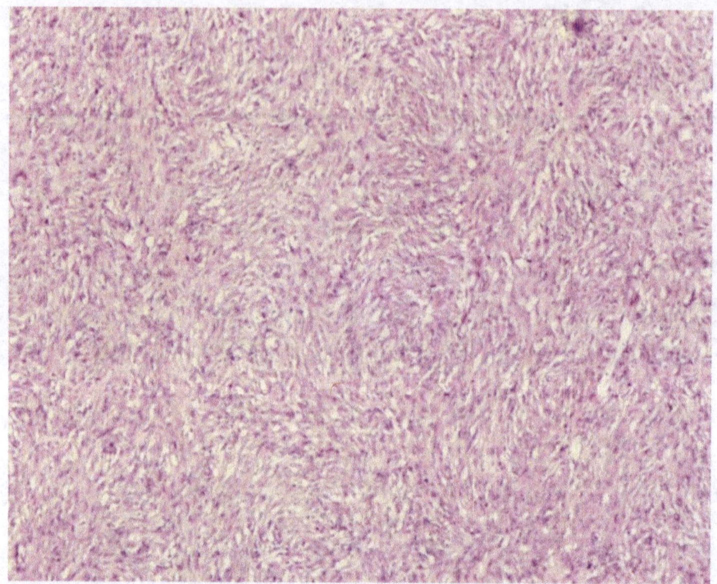

Fig. 63: Fibrosarcoma - Spindle shaped cells arranged in interwoven pattern with elongated to oval nuclei with eosinophilic cytoplasm H&E 4x

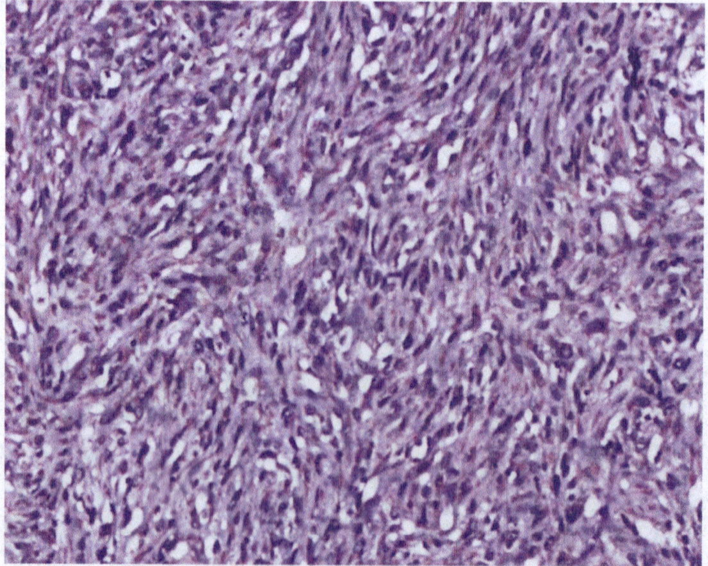

Fig. 64: Fibrosarcoma – Immunohistochemistry - Vimentin - Strong cytoplasmic signal 4x

33

Lipoma

Lipoma is a benign tumor of adipocytes and it is more common in dogs and mostly observed in the trunk, thigh and proximal limbs with rare presence of ulceration.

Grossly, the tumors reveal round (Figure 65) to soft light white to yellow color and upon incision, it is of greasy in consistency.

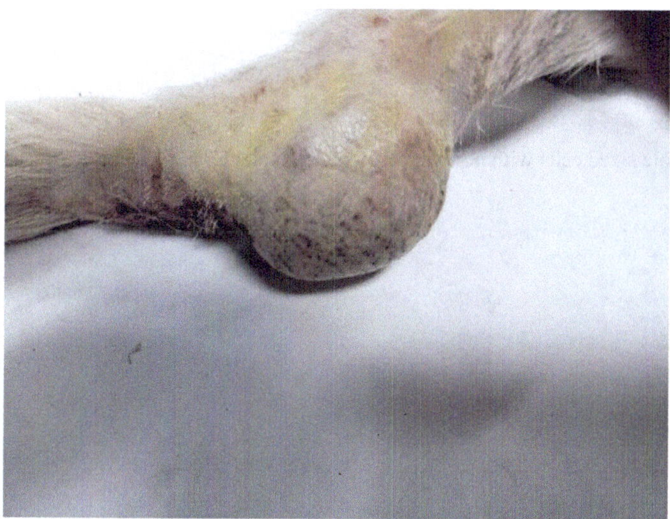

Fig. 65: Lipoma –Tail - Round, soft light white coloured nodule

Cytologically, round to spherical or polygonal shaped cells with thin rim of clear cytoplasm and peripherally located vacuolated area seen and the cells are mostly arranged as individual to clusters. It gives an oily appearance before getting dried up on a slide. It is usually acellular after dissolved by alcohol in Romanowsky stain.

Histopathologically, the neoplastic cells are identical to the variable sized adipocytes (Figure 66). Larger clear vacuoles with peripherally pushed nuclei are seen.

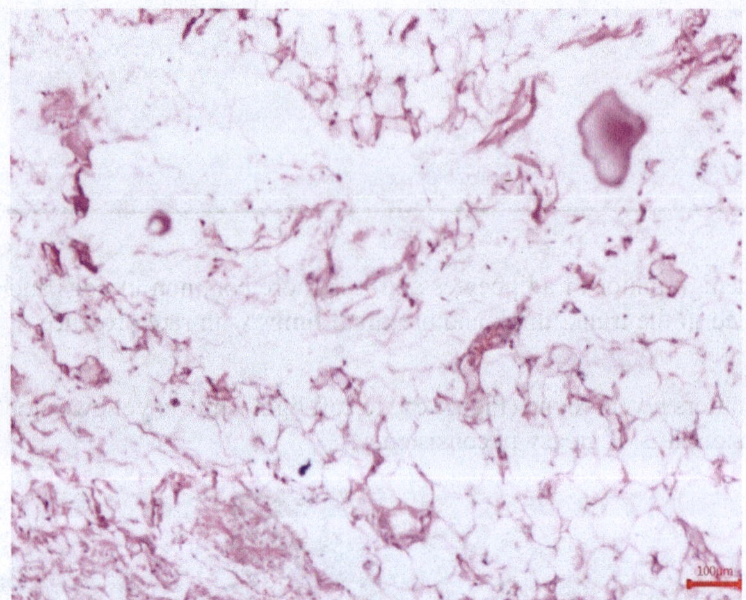

Fig. 66: Lipoma - Variable sized cells with peripherally pushed nuclei H&E Bar=100 µm

34

Liposarcoma

Liposarcoma is a rare malignant tumor of adipocytes in dogs.

Grossly, the neoplastic cells are arranged in less circumscribed to large firm to hard (Figure 67) nodules on the dermis and the nodules noticed on the subcutis are grey white in color.

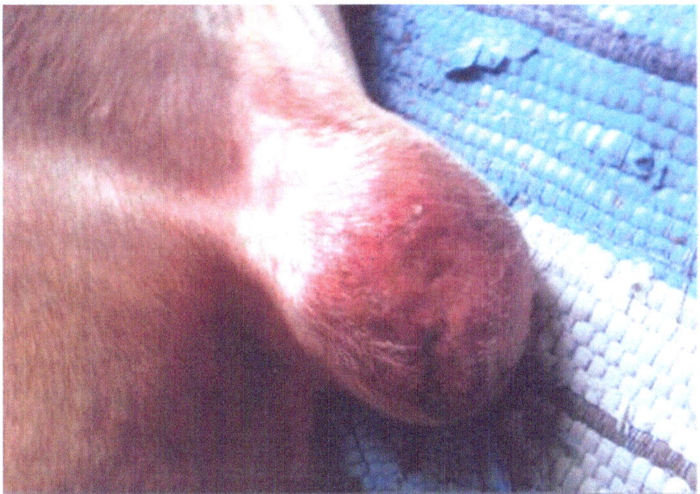

Fig. 67: Liposarcoma - Large firm mass above the right elbow in the lateral aspect

Cytologically, presence of moderate to high number of neoplastic cells arranged in individual or sheets is seen. Mostly, the cells are round to ovoid to spindloid shape and contain moderate to large round nuclei with varied pale cytoplasm. Cytoplasm also has vacuolations with peripherally placed nucleus. Mitotic figures are also seen.

Microscopically, neoplastic cells are round, polygonal, stellate or elongated cells with indistinct cell boundary with pale eosinophilic cytoplasm (Figure 68 & 69) and contain variable sized vacuoles, spherical vesicular nuclei and compressed cell membrane, single to multiple prominent nucleoli.

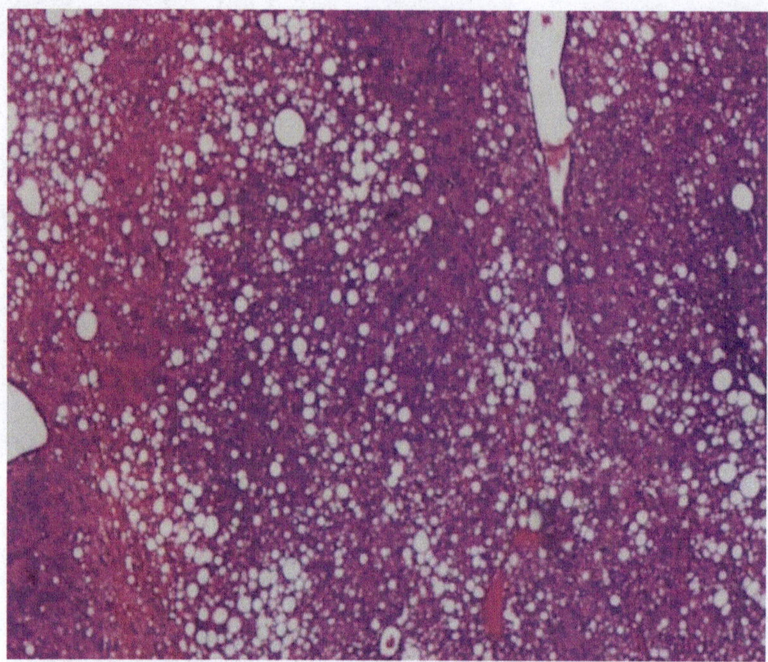

Fig. 68: Liposarcoma - Variable shaped cells with pale eosinophilic cytoplasm with spherical vesicular nuclei variable sized vacuoles H&E 10X

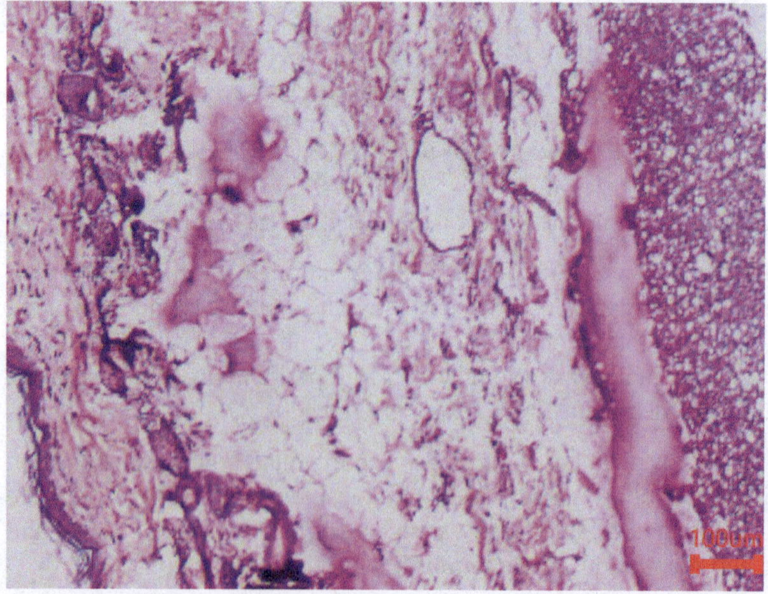

Fig. 69: Liposarcoma – Neoplastic foci in the subcutis H&E Bar=100 μm

35

Haemangioma

It is a benign tumor of endothelial cells. It is a common tumor of dogs. Solar induction is one of the cause for development of this tumor.

Grossly, lesions are well encapsulated nodules which are red to dark brown in colour.

Cytologically, hemangioma reveals oval, spindle to stellate shaped cells with moderate light basophilic cytoplasm and round or ovoid nucleus with smooth or fine lacy chromatin pattern and one or two small round indistinct nucleoli.

Histopathologically, neoplastic foci contain well circumscribed variable sized blood spaces filled with RBC (Figure 70) and lined by single layer of uniform endothelial cells in cavernous haemangioma.

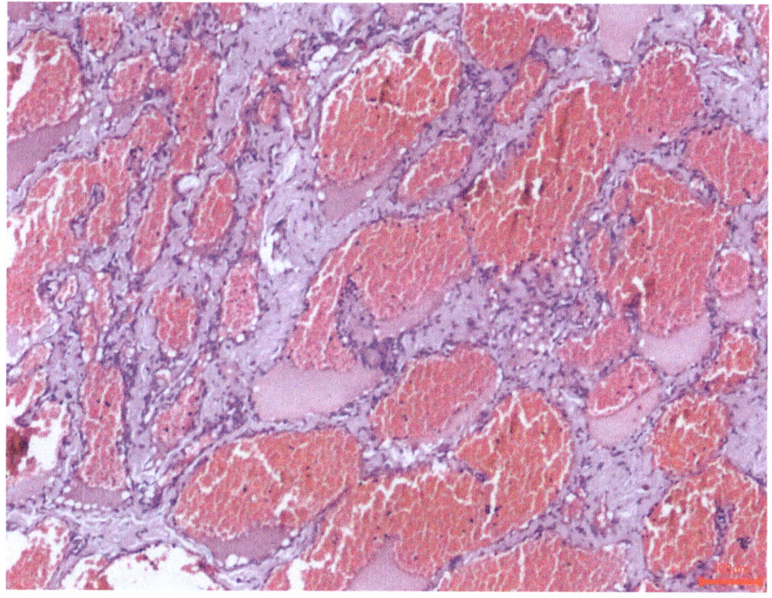

Fig. 70: Cavernous haemangioma - Variable sized large blood spaces filled with red blood cells H&E Bar=100 µm

36

Haemangiosarcoma

Haemangiosarcoma is a malignant tumour of vascular endothelial cells. It is more commonly seen in aged dogs.

Grossly, the tumors are soft to firm, round shaped red/ brown to black color which upon incision exude blood..

Cytology

On cytological examination, normal endothelial cells, medium to large sized cells (plumpy to spindle shaped cells), anisocytosis, anisokaryosis (round nuclei), prominent nucleoli and basophilic cytoplasm are seen. The cytological aspiration contains more blood.

Microscopically, numerous irregular immature anastomosing vascular channels separated by distinct collagen bundles in the dermis are seen. Variable sized plumpy neoplastic endothelial cells of spindle to polygonal to ovoid shaped with prominent pleomorphic hyperchromatic nuclei with more mitotic figures are seen. The presence of haemosiderin in macrophages is seen in the stroma.

37

Hemangiopericytoma

Hemangiopericytoma is a tumor originating from pericytes. It is mostly seen in distal extremities due to elevation of blood pressure in that area. It is mostly seen in skin and subcutaneous tissue around the joint region.

Grossly, solitary nodules, white, grey, red, soft to firm and rubbery to fatty in appearance are frequently seen.

Cytology reveals individual to small clusters of spindle shaped cells. It contains round or oval to caudate nuclei with moderate basophilic cytoplasm and stippled to reticulated chromatin. Some cells will be seen adhering to the surface of the capillary endothelial wall.

Histologically, the neoplastic masses show plumpy spindle shaped cells arranged in fingerprint (Figure 71) holes or interlacing bundles surrounding the vascular lumen

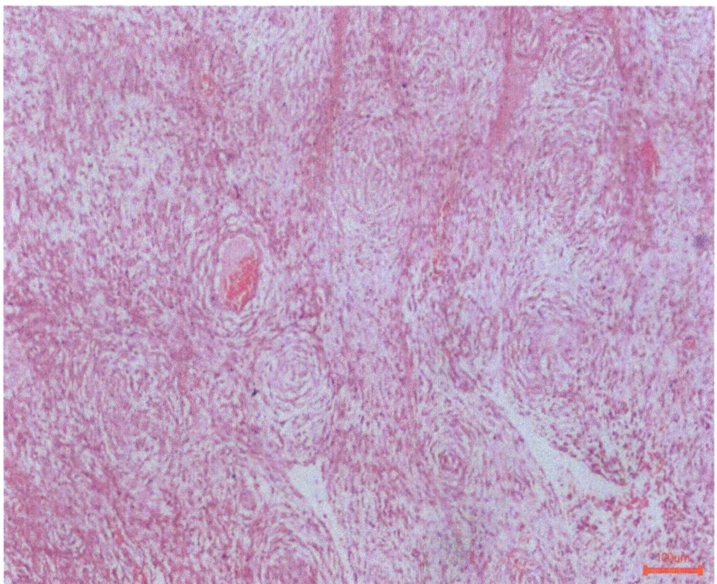

Fig. 71: Hemangiopericytoma - Plumpy spindle shaped cells arranged in finger print appearance around blood vessels H&E Bar=100 μm

Cutaneous Neoplasm – Round Cell Tumors

38

Mast Cell Tumour

The mast cell tumors are focal or multicentric in nature in the skin and occasionally in the internal organs. It is more common in middle aged dogs without sex predilection.

Gross pathology

Gross lesions reveal the neoplastic foci which are varied in appearance with light white (Figure 72) to yellow colour and consistency varied based on the degree of degranulation and secondary inflammation. In large tumors, ulceration is more common.

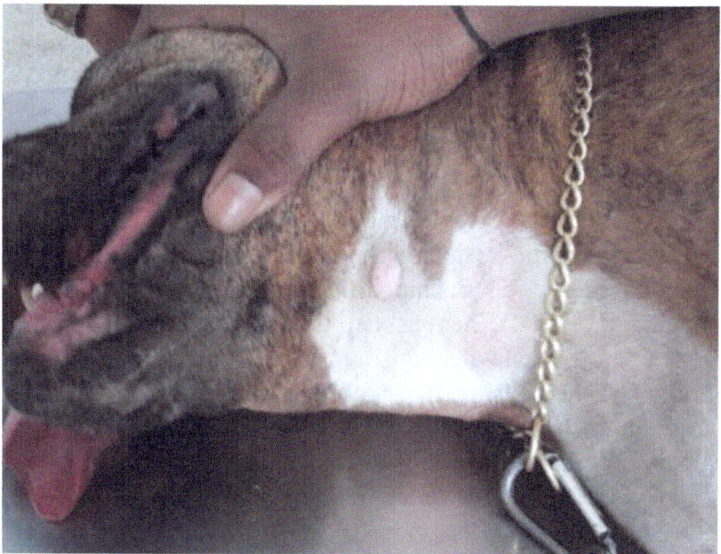

Fig. 72: Mast cell tumour - Single light white coloured nodule

Cytology reveals the presence of numerous neoplastic mast cells, high nuclear cytoplasmic ratio, pleomorphic hyperchromatic nuclei and cytoplasmic metachromatic granules (Figure 73). Cytoplasm is pale. Eosinophils are also seen.

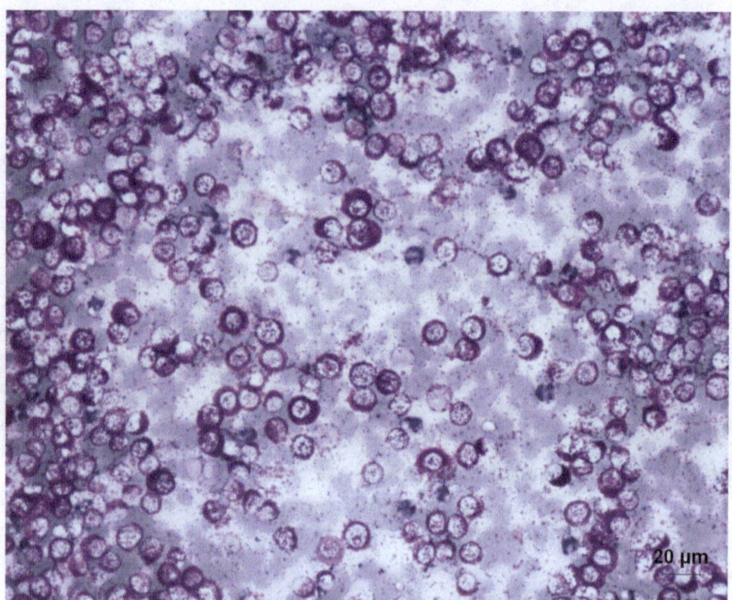

Fig. 73: Cytology-Mast cell tumour - Presence of numerous neoplastic mast cells, and cytoplasm contained purple granules. L&G Bar=20 µm

Histopathology

The microscopical examination reveals the presence of round to polygonal shaped neoplastic cells with centrally to slightly eccentrically placed round nuclei and moderate pale to pink cytoplasm containing granules having grey bluish granules (Figure 74). With the help of toluidine blue special stain, it will appear as purple colour (Figure 75). Eosinophilic infiltration is also observed. According to Patnaik *et al.* (1984), the mast cell tumours are categorized into three grades. Among them, grade I where the neoplastic foci seen in the dermis with intact epidermis and the cells are arranged in cords or sheets with grey blue cytoplasmic granules. It is well differentiated and highly granulated in the grade II mast cell tumours and not so well circumscribed when compared to grade I and it may get extended into deep dermis and subcutaneous tissue. Neoplastic cells are more pleomorphic, more sparsely granulated cytoplasm. In Grade III, poorly circumscribed mass with deep subcutis invasion, the cells are round to polyhedral or more pleomorphic cells in sheets to nest, large round vesicular nuclei, scanty to absent granules in the cytoplasm. CD117 (Figure 76) or C-Kit can be used for further confirmation by immunohistochemistry.

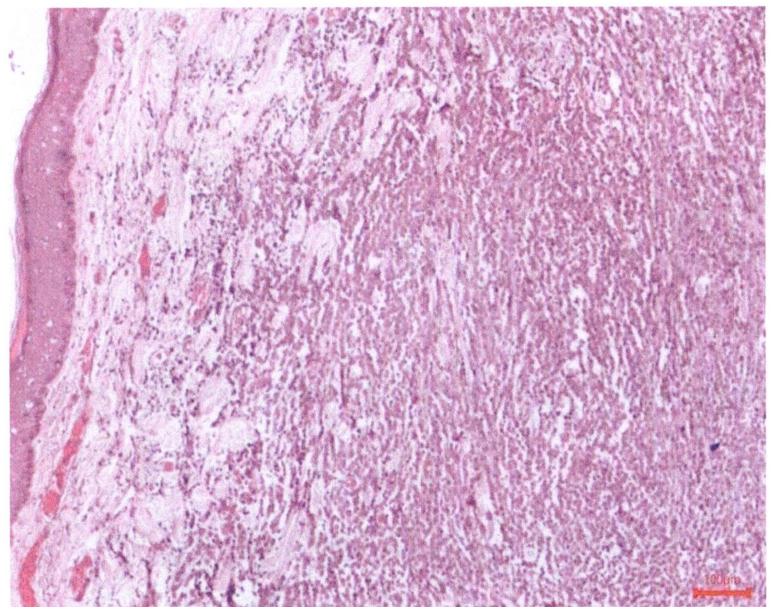

Fig. 74: Mast cell tumor - Round to polygonal cells containing round to oval nuclei with blue gray granules H&E Bar=100 µm

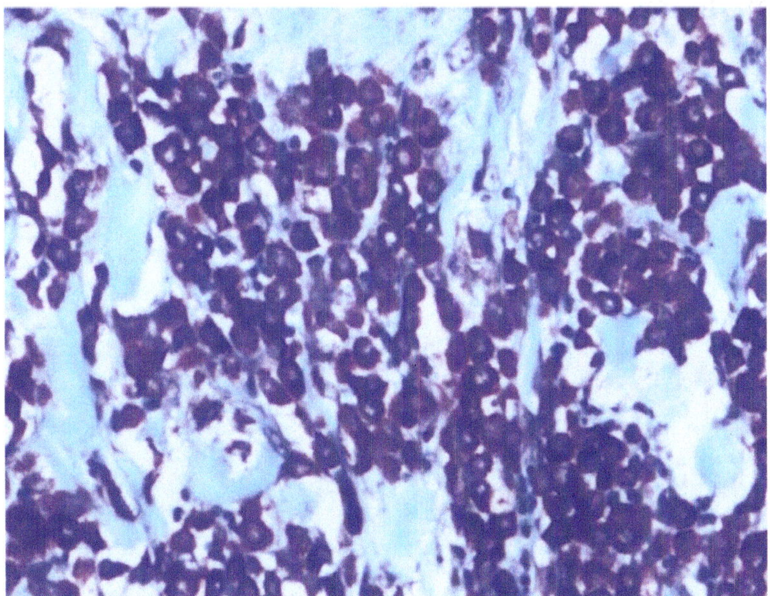

Fig. 75: Mast cell tumor - Purple coloured granules in the cytoplasm Toluidine blue stain 40x

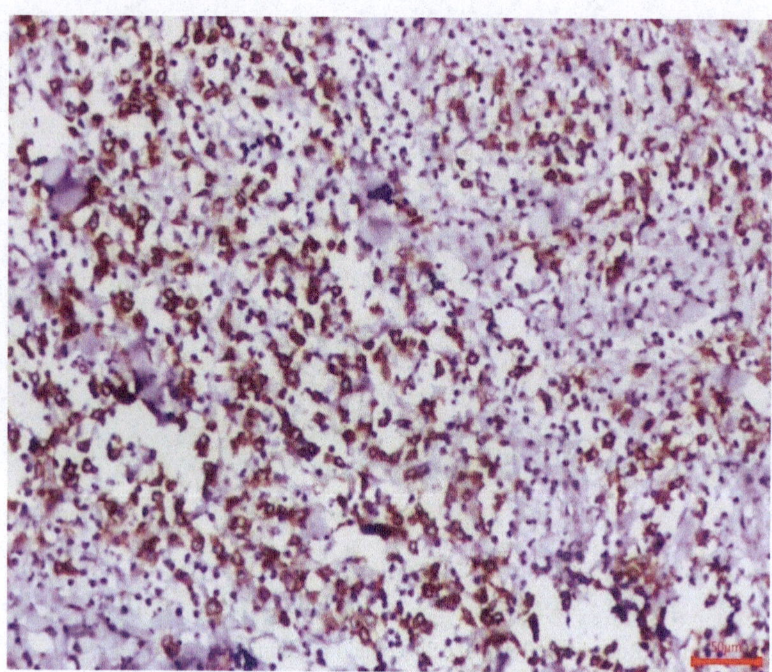

Fig. 76: Mast cell tumor - Immunohistochemistry - Strong brown coloured expression in the cytoplasm CD117 Bar=50 µm

39

Histiocytoma

Histiocytoma is more common in younger dogs below two years of age. It is also observed in all age groups.

Gross examination

Grossly, histiocytoma appears as light pink, smooth to firm, raised round (Figure 77) masses. Alopecia and ulceration are also observed.

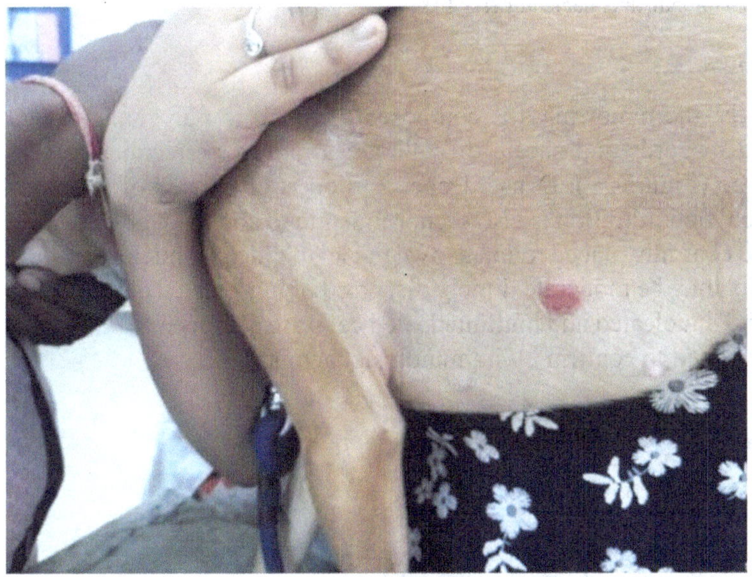

Fig. 77: Histiocytoma - Light pink, firm raised round mass

Cytologically, neoplastic cells are round in shape, with round to oval or ovoid indented (Figure 78) to cleaved nucleus and show indistinct nucleoli. Binucleation, multinucleation and nuclear moulding are also characteristic of histiocytoma.

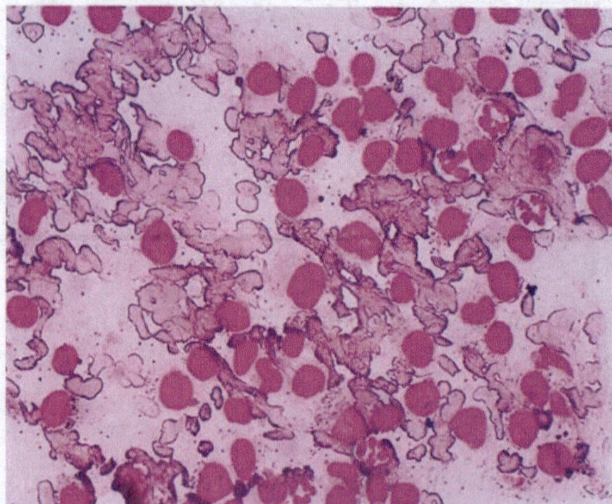

Fig. 78: Histiocytoma – Cytology - Round shaped, round to oval indented nucleus with indistinct nucleoli L&G 40X

Histopathology

Microscopically, the tumor mass is composed of round to polygonal shaped cells arranged in cords and sheets of cells are arranged perpendicularly to the skin surface (Figure 79). Dense deeper portion is composed of sheets of cells. Lymphocytic infiltration is also seen. Moderate to abundant eosinophilic cytoplasm and centrally placed round to oval nuclei to indented nuclei are seen. Mitotic activity may be moderate. Finely dispersed or marginated chromatin is seen in nuclei. Binucleated and multinucleated cells are also seen. CD18, CD1 and MHC2 are used to confirm by immunohistochemistry.

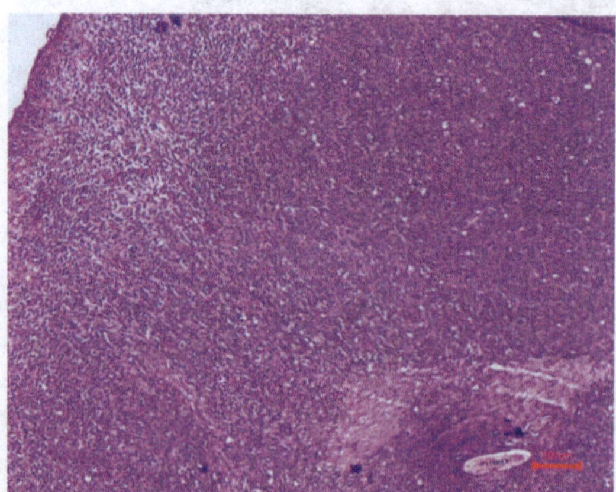

Fig. 79: Histiocytoma - Cords of neoplastic cells arranged perpendicular to skin surface H&E Bar=100 μm

40

Cutaneous Lymphoma (Mycosis Fungoides, Epitheliotropic T-Cell lymphoma)

Cutaneous lymphoma has two types *viz.* Epitheliotropic and non-epitheliotropic. Epitheliotropic lymphoma (mycosis fungoides) is mostly seen in the skin which is characterized by erythema, pruritus, alopecia, scaling, erosion and ulceration. It mostly occurs in plaques or nodules (Figure 80). Non-epitheliotropic lymphomas are observed as nodules. They are usually sheets of nodules seen in the deep dermal and subcutaneous tissue.

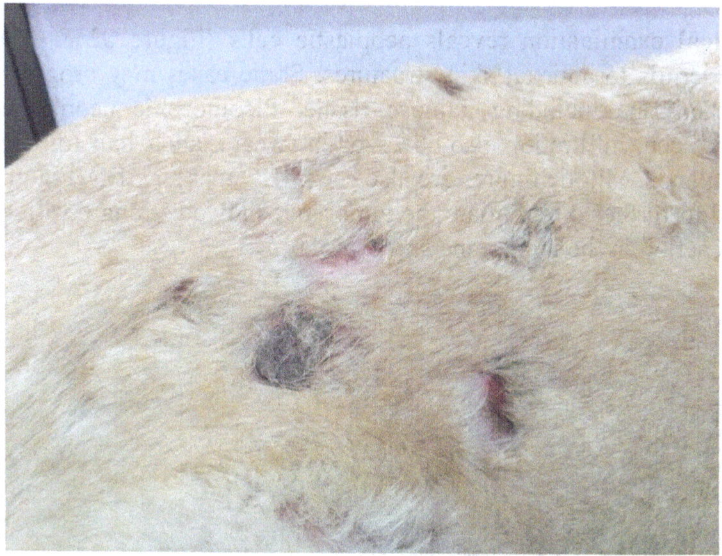

Fig. 80: Cutaneous lymphoma - Multiple nodules

Cytologically, presence of small to large sized lymphocytes with scanty to moderate basophilic cytoplasm are seen (Figure 81). Round to irregular indented nuclei is present in central to eccentric position which has ruptured to finely stippled chromatin is also noticed. Lymphoglandular bodies are also seen.

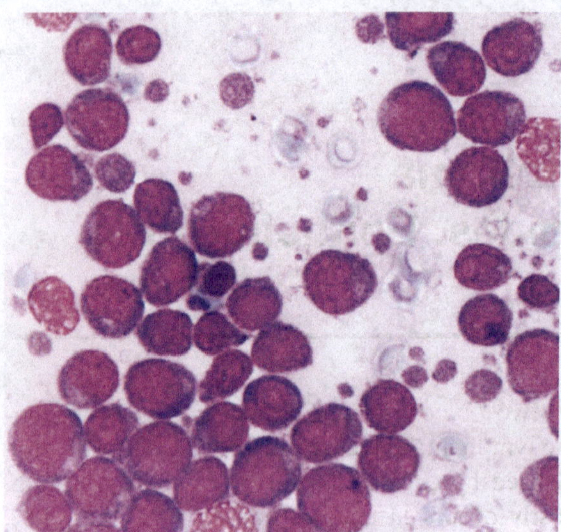

Fig. 81: Cytology- Lymphoma – Presence of variable sized lymphocytes with scanty basophilic cytoplasm and prominent multiple nucleoli. Lymphoglandular bodies were seen L&G 100X

Histopathological examination reveals neoplastic cells (Figure 82 & 83) seen in the epidermis to adnexal skin structures. Some cases may progress to subcutaneous tissue including adipose tissue. Pleomorphic neoplastic lymphocytes are seen. Infiltration also observed in sweat glands, hair follicle and sebaceous glands. Mitotic figures are also seen. IHC marker CD3 (Figure 84) can be used to further differentiate the tumor and showed strong positive brown colour reaction in the membrane and cytoplasm.

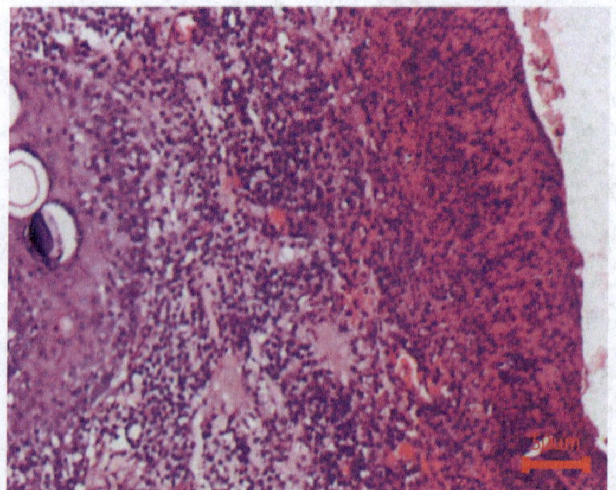

Fig. 82: Cutaneous T cell lymphoma - Clusters of neoplastic cells H&E Bar=50µm

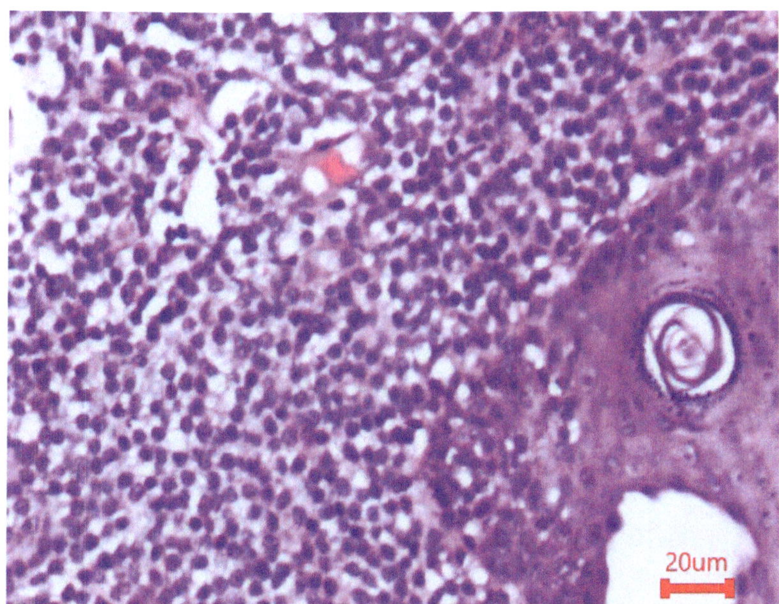

Fig. 83: T cell lymphoma - Clusters of neoplastic cells in the dermis H&E Bar=20 µm

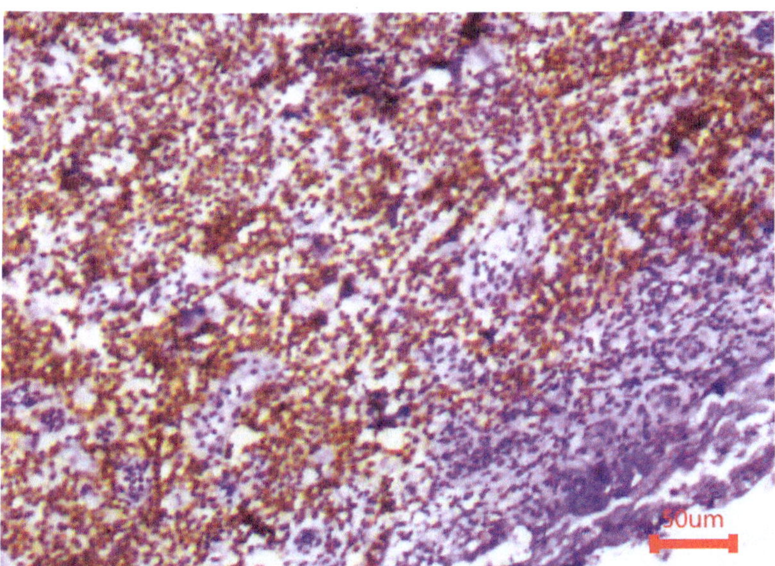

Fig. 84: T cell lymphoma – Immunohistochemistry - Strong positive brown colour reaction in the membrane and cytoplasm CD3 Bar=50 µm

41

Cutaneous Plasmacytoma

It is more common in old dogs and also mostly observed in the cutaneous region of trunk and legs.

Grossly, the tumour appears as solitary to multiple masses as white, pink to red, smooth, and raised nodules. Alopecia and ulceration are also observed. It is mostly observed in the pinna and digits.

Cytologically, the tumours reveal moderate to high cellularity, with large round eccentrically placed nucleus (Figure 85), coarse reticulated to stippled chromatin with indistinct nucleoli (some or few cells) and abundant blue cytoplasm with perinuclear halo. Binucleated cells are also seen. The nuclei are hyperchromatic.

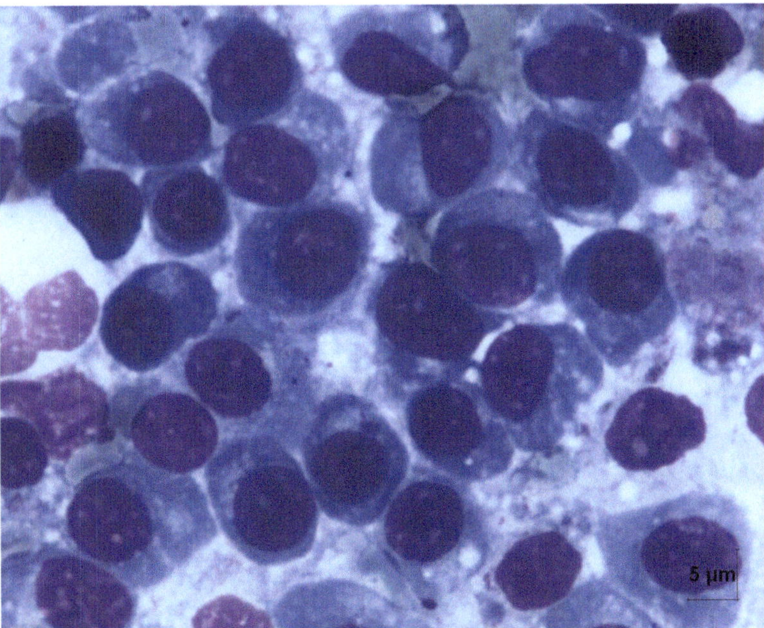

Fig. 85: Cytology-Plasmacytoma-Round cells with eccentrically placed hyperchromatic nucleus, coarse to stippled chromatin with indistinct nucleoli and abundant pale blue cytoplasm with perinuclear halo. L&G Bar=5 µm

Histopathologically, circumscribed single to multiple nodules which are non-encapsulated are seen in the dermis and in some cases, it may extend into the subcutis. Neoplastic cells are round to polygonal cells with eccentrically placed round to oval nucleus (Figure 86). Chromatin clumping is seen as cartwheel appearance. Perinuclear halo is also observed. The cytoplasm has either vacuoles or finely granular eosinophilic material and cells are arranged in clusters separated by fibrovascular stroma. Binucleated and multinucleated cells are also observed. Mitotic figures are also seen. CD138 and IgG lambda light chain are the specific markers for differentiation.

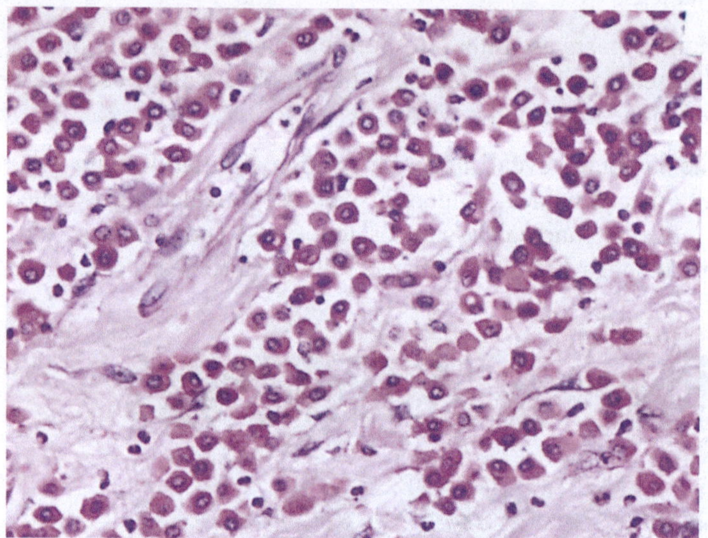

Fig. 86: Plasmacytoma - Round to polygonal cells with eccentrically placed round to oval nucleus H&E Bar=20µm

42

Melanoma

It is more common in dogs and frequently seen in the skin and oral cavity. It usually occurs in 5 to 11 years old dogs. Benign melanomas are solitary, circumscribed, alopecic firm and freely movable blue black coloured nodules in the skin. Malignant melanoma is sessile, polypoid to plaque like grey or brown black coloured granules in the skin with ulceration.

Grossly, tumours are irregular, solitary and circumscribed hard nodules which are black in colour.

Cytologically, numerous individual to clusters of cells are seen. Cells are round to stellate, spindle shaped with fine to moderate/brown to black coloured melanin granules in the cytoplasm (Figure 87). Sometimes, it may obscure the cytological details. Anisokaryosis and mitotic figures are commonly seen in malignant tumour.

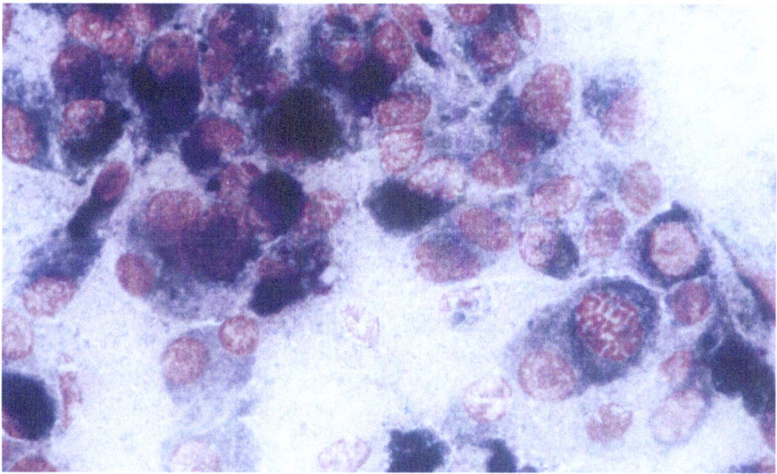

Fig. 87: Melanoma- Round to oval shaped cells with cytoplasm contained black granules Leishman &Giemsa x100 (Image Courtesy: Krithiga et al., 2005)

Histopathological examination reveals neoplastic cells of round, polygonal, spindle, epithelioidal in shape or in combination. Among them, spindle and epithelioid combination are more common. The cells are arranged in nest or holes pattern or sometimes arranged in the form of sheets. The cells are round to polygonal shape and are separated by scanty fibrous connective tissue stroma. Slightly elongated round to oval nuclei and vesicular nuclei with small or inconspicuous nucleoli are seen. Black coloured melanin pigment granules are seen in cytoplasm (Figure 88). Sometimes, it may completely mask the cell. Fontana Masson's silver impregnation method is used to identify melanin pigment. Malignant melanoma is composed of predominantly non pigmented spindle, round to polygonal or epithelioidal cells, moderate to marked nuclear pleomorphism and prominent nucleoli with high mitotic rate of 3 to more.

It should be confirmed by immunohistochemistry using S100 and MelanA..

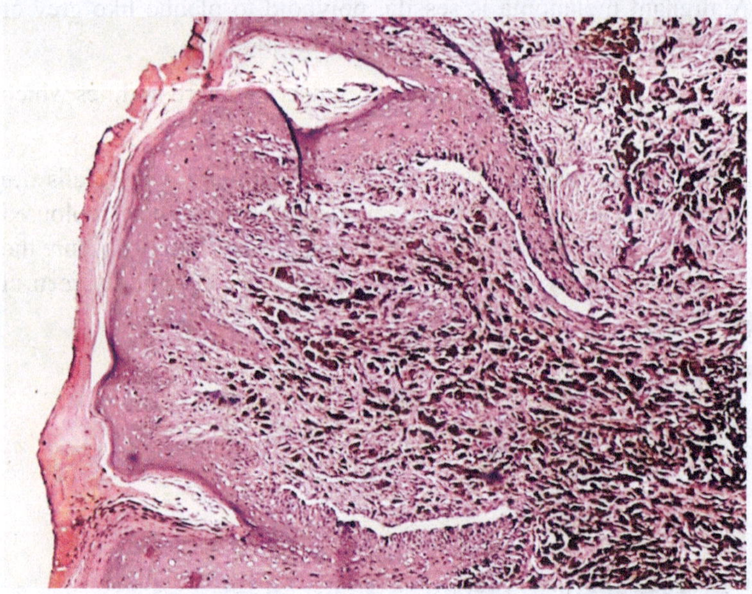

Fig. 88: Melanoma – Dermis - Round to polygonal shaped cells containing brown black pigments H&E Bar=100 µm

43

Transmissible Venereal Tumour (Sticker Tumour, Canine Venereal Granuloma)

It is commonly spread by coitus and also by licking and rubbing of the affected area. It is more common in active breeding dogs.

Grossly, the tumour manifests as single to multilobulated masses. The surface is ulcerated (Figure 89) and friable. Some may be smooth or granular. It is of variable size.

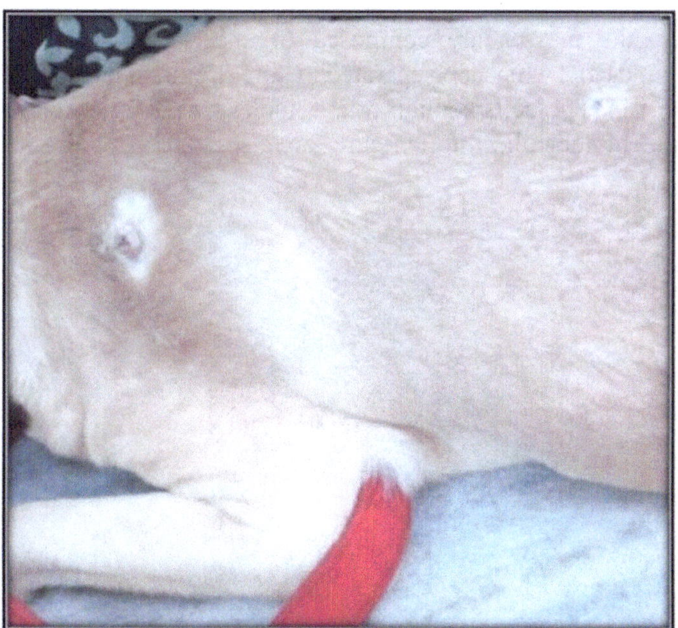

Fig. 89: Transmissible venereal tumour - Nodular type, ulcerated

Cytological examination reveals the presence of numerous round cells with round to oval centrally placed nuclei containing delicate chromatin and one or two prominent nucleoli. Cytoplasm also contains distinct clear vacuoles (Figure 90).

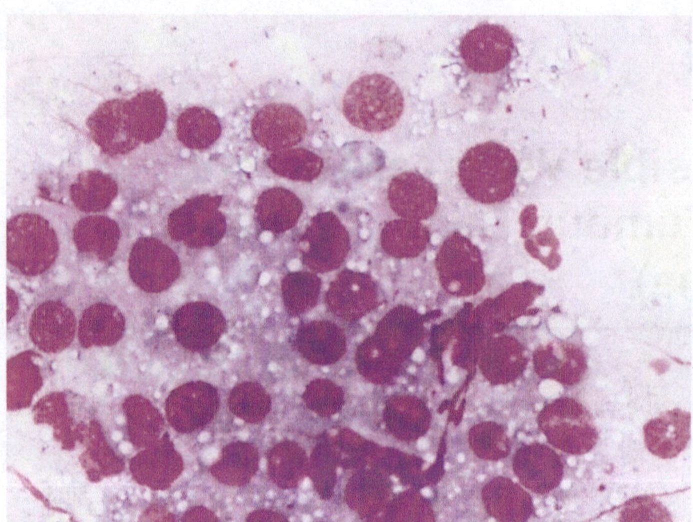

Fig. 90: Cytology -Transmissible venereal tumour - Round cells with central nuclei and vacuolated cytoplasm L&G 40X

Histopathologically, the masses are composed of sheets and cords of neoplastic cells of round cells which are separated by fine stroma in the dermis and subcutis (Figure 91). The cells contain round nuclei with fine to coarse chromatin and prominent nucleoli. Mitotic figures are also seen.

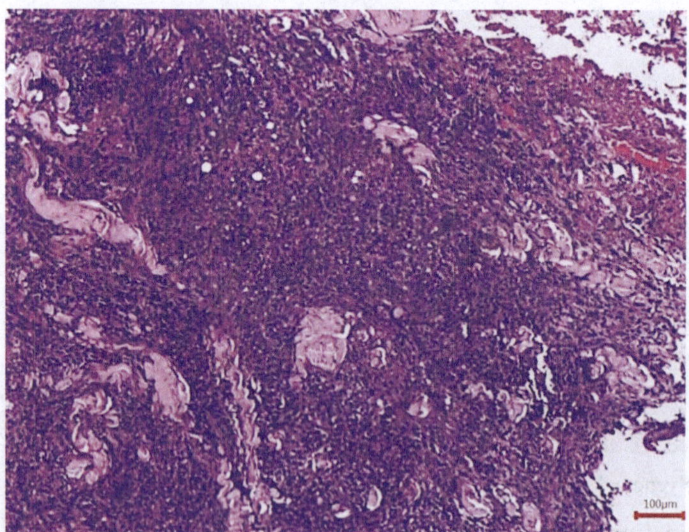

Fig. 91: Transmissible venereal tumour - Sheets and cords of round cells with fine stroma in the dermis and subcutis H&E Bar=100μm.

References

Cowell, R.L., Tyler, R.D., Meinkoth, J.H. and DeNicola, D.B. (2008). Diagnostic Cytology and Hematology of the Dog and Cat. Third Edition, Mosby Elsevier, Missouri, USA

Gross, T.L., Ihrke, P.J., Walder, E.J. and Affolter, V.K. (2005). Skin Diseases of the Dog and Cat: Clinical and Histopathologic Diagnosis. 2nd Edition, Blackwell Publishing Company, Ames, Iowa, USA

Meuten, D.J. (2002). Tumors in Domestic Animals. Fourth Edition, Wiley India Private Ltd., New Delhi, India

Raskin, R.E. and Meyer,D.J. (2010). Canine and Feline Cytology. AColor Atlas and Interpretation Guide. Second Edition, Saunders Elsevier, Missouri, USA

Yager, J.A. and Wilcock, B.P.(1994). Color Atlas and Text of Surgical Pathology of the Dog and Cat. Dermatopathology and skin tumors. Wolfe Publishing, UK.

Zachary, J.F. (2017). Pathologic Basis of Veterinary Disease. Sixth Edition, Elsevier, Missouri, USA.

Index